CLINICAL RHEUMATOLOGY

Second Edition

FUNDAMENTAL AND CLINICAL ASPECTS OF INTERNAL MEDICINE

A Series of Volumes for the Postgraduate Course

THE UNIVERSITY OF MIAMI SCHOOL OF MEDICINE
Department of Internal Medicine
William J. Harrington, M.D., Chairman
Jose S. Bocles, M.D., Coordinator

PUBLISHED

MEDICAL ONCOLOGY
Howard E. Lessner, M.D., Editor

CLINICAL RHEUMATOLOGY
Second Edition
John H. Talbott, M.D., Editor

FUNDAMENTAL AND CLINICAL ASPECTS OF INTERNAL MEDICINE
A Series of Volumes for the Postgraduate Course

CLINICAL RHEUMATOLOGY

Second Edition

Edited by
JOHN H. TALBOTT, M.D.
THE UNIVERSITY OF MIAMI SCHOOL OF MEDICINE
Department of Internal Medicine
William J. Harrington, M.D., Chairman
Jose S. Bocles, M.D., Coordinator

ELSEVIER • NEW YORK
New York • Oxford

Elsevier North Holland, Inc.
52 Vanderbilt Avenue, New York, New York 10017

Sole distributors outside the United States and Canada:

Elsevier Science Publishers, B.V.
P.O. Box 211, 1000 AE Amsterdam, The Netherlands

Library of Congress Cataloging in Publication Data

Main entry under title:

Clinical rheumatology.
(Fundamental and clinical aspects of internal medicine)

Includes bibliographical references and index.
1. Rheumatism. I. Talbott, John Harold, 1902–
II. Series. [DNLM: 1. Arthritis. 2. Rheumatism.
WE 544 C641]
RC927.C54 1981 616.7'23 81-5371
ISBN 0-444-00615-X AACR2
ISBN 0-444-00634-6 (pbk.)

Manufactured in the United States of America

Contributing Authors

ROY D. ALTMAN, M.D.

WILBUR J. BLECHMAN, M.D.

HARVEY E. BROWN, M.D.

NORMAN L. GOTTLIEB, M.D.

DAVID S. HOWELL, M.D.

FRED H. HYER, M.D.

JOHN J. JENNINGS, M.D.

JULIO C. PITA, Ph.D.

DUANE R. SCHULTZ, Ph.D.

JOHN H. TALBOTT, M.D.

HAL B. UNSCHULD, M.D.

J. F. WOESSNER, Jr., Ph.D.

CONTENTS

GENERAL PREFACE TO THE SECOND EDITION ix

EDITOR'S PREFACE xi

THE COMPLEMENT SYSTEM AND INFLAMMATION
Duane R. Schultz, Ph.D. 1

SEROLOGY / Duane R. Schultz, Ph.D. 20

MEDIATORS OF THE INFLAMMATORY PROCESS
Duane R. Schultz, Ph.D. 28

SYNOVIANALYSIS / Norman L. Gottlieb, M.D. 41

RHEUMATOID ARTHRITIS / Norman L. Gottlieb, M.D. 51

JUVENILE RHEUMATOID ARTHRITIS
Wilbur J. Blechman, M.D. 66

ANKYLOSING SPONDYLITIS / Harvey E. Brown, M.D. 73

PSORIATIC ARTHRITIS / David S. Howell, M.D. 79

FELTY'S SYNDROME / David S. Howell, M.D. 83

SJÖGREN'S SYNDROME / Harvey E. Brown, M.D. 85

REITER'S SYNDROME / Norman L. Gottlieb, M.D. 87

VIRAL ARTHRITIS
Fred H. Hyer, M.D. and Norman L. Gottlieb, M.D. 93

LYME DISEASE
Hal B. Unschuld, M.D., and Norman L. Gottlieb, M.D. 98

SYSTEMIC LUPUS ERYTHEMATOSUS / Roy D. Altman, M.D. 102

ACUTE DERMATOMYOSITIS-POLYMYOSITIS
John H. Talbott, M.D. 112

POLYARTERITIS / Norman L. Gottlieb, M.D. 118

SCLERODERMA (PROGRESSIVE SYSTEMIC SCLEROSIS)
Roy D. Altman, M.D. 123

MIXED CONNECTIVE TISSUE DISEASE
John H. Talbott, M.D. 130

EOSINOPHILIC FASCIITIS / John H. Talbott, M.D. 132

POLYMYALGIA RHEUMATICA / John H. Talbott, M.D. 134

ACUTE RHEUMATIC FEVER / John H. Talbott, M.D. 136

GONOCOCCAL ARTHRITIS / Roy D. Altman, M.D. 141

JOINT DISEASE IN SARCOIDOSIS / John H. Talbott, M.D. 146

PURINE METABOLISM / Julio C. Pita, Ph.D. 147

GOUT AND HYPERURICEMIA / John H. Talbott, M.D. 152

PATHOPHYSIOLOGY OF CARTILAGE
J. F. Woessner, Jr., Ph.D. 163

OSTEOARTHRITIS / David S. Howell, M.D. 172

LOW BACKACHE / David S. Howell, M.D. 181

BURSITIS, TENDONITIS, AND FIBROSITIS
Wilbur J. Blechman, M.D. 184

CHONDROCALCINOSIS / David S. Howell, M.D. 187

HEMOCHROMATOSIS / Roy D. Altman, M.D. 190

OCHRONOSIS / Norman L. Gottlieb, M.D. 193

PAGET'S DISEASE / Roy D. Altman, M.D. 198

TOTAL JOINT REPLACEMENT / John J. Jennings, M.D. 207

INDEX 213

GENERAL PREFACE TO THE SECOND EDITION

Six years ago the Department of Internal Medicine of the University of Miami School of Medicine inaugurated an annual series of post-graduate courses entitled "Fundamental and Clinical Aspects of Internal Medicine." The first course, prompted by many requests from area physicians and medical societies, was timed to precede by one to two weeks the initial recertification examination of the American Board of Internal Medicine.

Among the teaching materials developed for this course was a group of booklets designed to follow or to implement the lecture presentations of subject matter judged to be most pertinent to internists qualified for certification. Since the course was intensive and of two weeks duration only, we realized that the subsequent matter to be presented had to be carefully selected, with assumptions made concerning content presumed to be already well known and also concerning material that would not in our judgment be needed by a competent general internist, although of great importance to the subspecialist.

The course has now been given in each of the past six years. Its quality has been widely noted, and many physicians both from the United States and other countries have become annual registrants. Accordingly, it was believed that the course booklets might find a wider appeal if they were professionally produced and distributed by a publisher. This objective has been concluded by an agreement with Elsevier North Holland to publish the series.

It should be stressed that these volumes are not intended to be comprehensive. They do not cover subject matter in the breadth ordinarily found in standard textbooks or monographs, but rather they supplement standard teaching materials. In order to be useful for the review course, these compilations are inexpensive and are revised and updated periodically to maintain currency with advances in their respective areas.

We acknowledge the immeasurable help of our staff coordinator, Mrs. Arlene Gunn, the several members of the secretarial staff of the divisions who contributed to the preparation of these volumes, and the organizational talents of the editors of each of the series.

JOSE S. BOCLES, M.D.
WILLIAM J. HARRINGTON, M.D.

EDITOR'S PREFACE

For more than a decade, the members of the Faculty of Medicine in the Department of Rheumatology at the University of Miami School of Medicine have prepared manuscripts on the subjects of their particular interest prior to presentation, either to undergraduate students or to symposia sponsored by the Postgraduate Division of the Department of Internal Medicine. The contents of each chapter are revised and updated annually and reviewed by the Editorial Committee before dissemination. The final drafts of the most recent reviews comprise these presentations for the second edition of *Clinical Rheumatology.*

Since most of the students in the various stages of learning just noted, irrespective of age, are essentially nonrheumatologists, these presentations have been designed to appeal to such categories and to fill an obvious void. In the final analysis, however, it can be stated without fear of contradiction that each of us, teacher, student, or postgraduate participant, is eager to learn, since the field of rheumatology is rapidly progressing and full of innovations in contrast to early in this century when progress was similar to the pace of the proverbial snail.

This volume provides a concise description of the clinical aspects of each of the important rheumatic conditions, with particular interest in the various forms and subleties of clinical subsets and clinical findings, as well as the vagaries of therapy.

Except for gout and osteoarthritis (degenerative joint disease), and a smattering of information regarding atrophic arthritis (rheumatoid arthritis) and its variants, most of the information contained herein was born in my lifetime. Even the terms in association with some joint diseases that might well have existed but were unrecognized centuries ago are recent. But a few of the recent terms might be mentioned:

Reiter's disease, polymyalgia rheumatica, chondrocalcinosis, Whipple's disease, sarcoidosis, systemic lupus erythematosus, eosinophilic fasciitis, Lyme arthritis, mixed connected tissue disease, and certain types of necrotizing vasculitis. In keeping with the proliferation of specific entities is the progress in development of diagnostic procedures and tests of the various types of joint disease. Thus the RA factor, the several histocompatibility antigens but especially the HLA-B27, and the significance of the complement system, all extremely valuable procedures in the diagnosis of specific types of joint disease, have been discovered in this generation.

The references listed after each subject have been selected because of the comprehensive nature or contemporary pertinence. Extended bibliographies in the chapters on the Complement System and Inflammation and the Mediators of the Inflammatory Process are justified because of the many recent advances in these areas.

For the student who wants additional information, expanded discussions of several features of the rheumatic diseases may be found in the following examples of comprehensive treatises that have been published recently.

Kelley WN, Harris ED Jr. Ruddy S, Sledge CB. Textbook of Rheumatology. Philadelphia: Saunders, 1981, Vol. 2.

Cohen AS. Rheumatology in Immunology. New York: Grune & Stratton, 1979.

McCarty DJ. Arthritis and Allied Conditions. Philadelphia: Lea & Febiger, 9th ed, 1979.

The Arthritis Division is deeply indebted to Mr. and Mrs. Paul Frohring and to Mrs. William L. McKnight for their support of the several division activities, including the preparation of this volume.

JOHN H. TALBOTT, M.D.
Coordinator for Teaching
Arthritis Division

CLINICAL RHEUMATOLOGY

Second Edition

THE COMPLEMENT SYSTEM AND INFLAMMATION

DUANE R. SCHULTZ, PhD.

Activation of the complement (C) proteins in plasma and other biologic fluids represents an important amplifying system for producing tissue damage in many of the connective tissue diseases (1–9). Thus the majority of these diseases have at least one feature in common: an *immunologically induced inflammation* in which C is one of the major effectors.

There are two major C pathways: the classic pathway and the alternative or properdin pathway.[1] The components of the classic pathway may be divided into (1) a recognition unit, C1 (C1q, C1r, C1s held together with calcium); (2) the two natural substrates of C$\overline{1}$[2], which together form a C3-converting unit (C4, C2); (3) the C3 component that is common to both pathways; and (4) the membrane attack unit C5, C6, C7, C8, and C9. The alternative pathway bypasses the early-acting C1, C4, and C2 steps, but it includes both native C3 and its activated form, namely C3b. Like the classic pathway, the alternative pathway also may lead to the activation of C5 to C9. It is the mechanism of native C3 conversion that differentiates the two pathways. Both inhibitors and inactivators found in normal plasma and at least two divalent cations, i.e., calcium and magnesium in the classic pathway and magnesium in the alternative pathway, comprise the *complement system* (Fig. 1).

---

[1]Many different investigators have contributed information for the formulation of the C pathways. It is not possible to include all the individual reports in a review of this magnitude. Most of the individual contributions are cited in the comprehensive reviews in references 1–9.

[2]Activated C components may be designated with a bar over a number or letter (e.g., C$\overline{1}$) or by a lowercase letter (e.g., B $\rightarrow$ Ba + Bb).

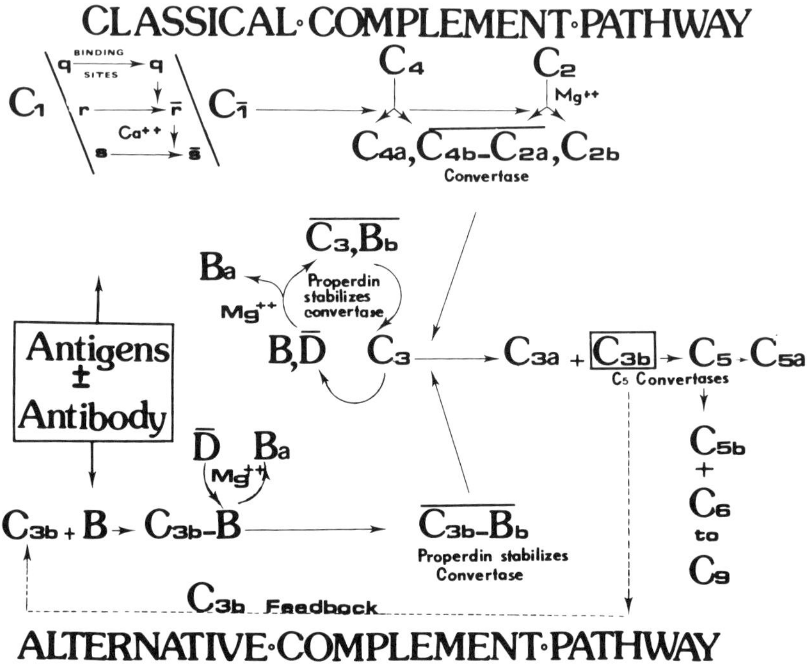

FIGURE 1

The components and metal cations of the classic and alternative (properdin) complement pathways. A bar over a number or letter (e.g., C$\bar{1}$) indicates that the component is activated. Both pathways do not require antibody for activation. Capital letters and arabic numbers are used for individual proteins, and small letters for cleavage products.

Additional factors control the biologic activities of the pathways. The anaphylatoxic fragments that originate from native C3 and C5, as well as bradykinin from the kallikrein system, are controlled by a normal plasma enzyme with carboxypeptidase-B-like activity, called the anaphylatoxin inactivator. A single cleavage of the COOH-terminal arginine of these phlogistic peptides is the mechanism of action (10). In addition, the chemotactic properties of the fragment C5a and the complex C$\overline{567}$ are inactivated by two factors with enzymatic activity in normal human plasma. The factors are unlike the anaphylatoxin inactivator (11).

Immunoglobulins have an important role in the activation of the classic C pathway. Characteristically, the plasma and other biologic fluids of patients with diseases such as rheumatoid arthritis (RA) and systemic lupus erythematosus (SLE) often contain antibodies to a number of self-antigens. Immunochemical studies of RA have concentrated on antiimmunoglobulins, just as those of SLE have centered on antibodies directed against various autologous nuclear components from, for example, both DNA and RNA, blood cells, anticoagulants, and cardiolipin. These autoantibodies together with C may produce disease directly, as with the extravascular or intravascular hemolysis of red cells in autoimmune hemolytic anemia, or indirectly, as in the acute glomerulonephritis caused by circulating, soluble antigen-antibody complexes that become lodged in glomeruli. It seems likely that antigen-antibody complexes also play a major role in polyarthritis and some forms of chronic liver disease.

The immunoglobulin classes that most commonly activate the classic C pathway are IgG (subclasses IgG1, IgG2, IgG3; but not IgG4) and IgM (both 19S and 7S). In arthritis, rheumatoid factors (RF) are antibodies against the patient's gammaglobulins, usually of the IgM class, but IgG and IgA have been described. The major specificity of the antibody is directed toward determinants on the patient's own IgG molecules. Because RF-IgG complexes may activate C, this reaction has phlogistic importance in the pathogenesis of RA. The reactive sites on these immunoglobulin molecules for C activation are on the Fc portion of the heavy chains [the fragment (F) of heavy chains that crystalizes (c) readily when separated from the native immunoglobulin molecule].

The alternative C pathway often is described as providing natural defense against microbial infection independent of antibody, whereas classic pathway activation depends on antigen-antibody complexes or aggregated immunoglobulin (8). This viewpoint is no longer tenable because there are a number of reports describing classic C pathway activation in the absence of antibodies. In brief, the lipid A component of bacterial endotoxin (12), some RNA viruses (13), certain bacteria (14), and some polysaccharides (15) cause activation of the classic C pathway independent of antigen-antibody complexes. Thus both pathways may provide a natural defense against microbes in the absence of antibody. Detailed discussions of autoimmune processes in RA and their role in pathogenesis are found elsewhere (16,17).

CLASSIC COMPLEMENT PATHWAY

The classic C pathway (Fig. 1) is initiated after trimolecular C1 binds to antigen-antibody complexes via the C1q portion of the molecule. C1q has six globular heads connected by six strands to a central core (5). These heads bind to the Fc portion of IgG or IgM. Following the

FIGURE 2

Activation and cleavage of native C3 via the classic and alternative complement pathway convertases. The fragments C3a and C3b from the initial cleavage of C3 are depicted, as well as the enzymatic degradation of C3b to the fragments C3c, C3d, and C3e by the C3b inactivator, by β_1H globulin, and by other proteases. Also shown are the biological activities of the various fragments.

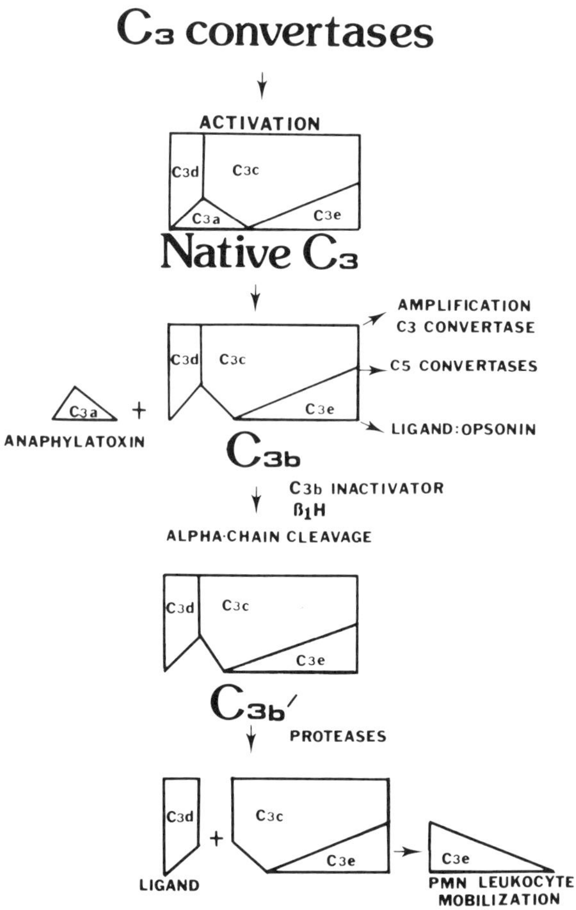

attachment, C1r (a serine protease) is activated, possibly because of an internal rearrangement, and C1s (a serine protease) is proteolytically cleaved to an activated form. Although antigen-antibody complexes are perhaps the major mechanism for activating C1 in connective tissue diseases, other tissue and humoral enzymes such as trypsin and plasmin, lysosomal proteases, and nonenzymic factors (see earlier) are capable of this function. The C1q portion of C1 is of interest chemically because the six connecting strands on the molecule and the central core have a composition similar to that of collagen. Following activation of C1, the next steps involve the two natural substrates for this component, C4 and C2.

A fragment is cleaved and released during the process of C4 activation (C4a) and C2 activation (C2b). Magnesium is required for the action of $C\overline{1}$ on C2. Activated C4 (C4b) combines with activated C2 (C2a) to form the next enzymic intermediary in the sequence, $C\overline{4b,2a}$. The latter is termed the classic pathway C3 convertase because it activates the next component in the sequence, C3. The activation of C3 and its cleavage products are shown in Figure 2. This reaction is perhaps one of the most significant in the cascade because cellbound

FIGURE 3

Pictorial representation of receptor sites for complement fragments C3b and C3d on a phagocytic cell membrane. The fragments are shown on red blood cells (RBC) sensitized with "Y-shaped" antibodies. The specific binding of the red cells to the phagocytic cell membrane receptors via C3b and C3d results in enhanced phagocytosis.

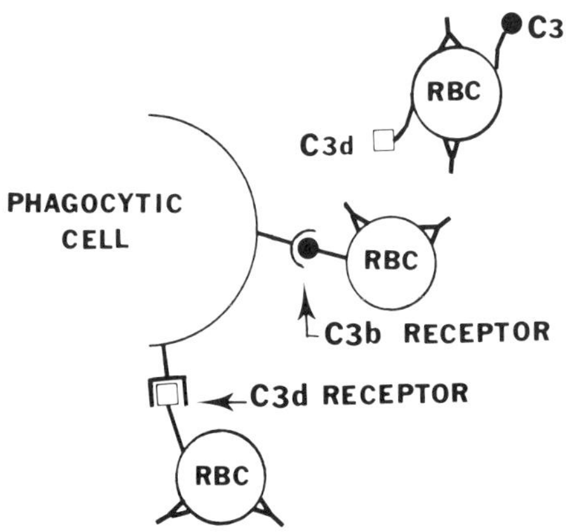

C3b (C3c, C3d, C3e) promotes adherence of erythrocytes, platelets, bone marrow-derived (B) lymphocytes, and phagocytic cells to receptor sites on other cells (immune adherence). In addition, after C3b and/or one of its fragments (C3d) are bound to receptor sites on microbial agents, red cells, and other antigens sensitized with antibody, the phagocytic processes of adherence and ingestion are enhanced (Fig. 3). A portion of C3c, termed C3e, causes PMN leukocyte mobilization (6). C3a, a small fragment released in the initial cleavage of C3, is an anaphylatoxin and is one of the most potent enhancers of capillary permeability.

Following the cleavage of native C3, C3b binds to $\overline{\text{C4b,2a}}$ to form a C5 convertase $\overline{\text{C4b,2a,3b}}$. The latter cleaves native C5 to C5a and C5b. C5a is a small molecular weight fragment that is a potent chemotactic factor. In addition, it causes an increase in capillary permeability and has anaphylatoxic activity. Both C3a and C5a have been isolated directly from RA lesions. C5b binds to C6, then to C7, and the $\overline{\text{C5b,6,7}}$ complex is also capable of promoting chemotaxis. In addition, this complex may bind to cell membranes, so-called bystander cells, and then accepts the two terminal components C8 and C9. A concentration-dependent lysis occurs after C8 is bound. C9 promotes the final disruption of the membrane if these sequential reactions occur on a cell surface. The C5b to C9 complex in a dimer form now resembles the "doughnutlike" structure that has been observed on a number of different cellular membranes in the electron microscope, including blood cells, bacteria, and viruses. This structure is responsible for the ultimate lysis of the cell, but the mechanism is still under investigation (2,5,6).

It is emphasized that the final lytic process requires the function of most of the C components acting sequentially, whereas the effectors of inflammation are mediated by the earlier-acting cleavage products C3a, C5a, $\overline{\text{C5b,6,7}}$, and Ba (see following).

ALTERNATIVE COMPLEMENT PATHWAY

The second major C pathway, the alternative or properdin pathway, bypasses C1, C4 and C2 (18). It also is detailed in Figure 1. Activation is initiated by aggregated immunoglobulins (notably IgA), polysaccharides, lipopolysaccharides, and other factors. Conceptually, the pathway was thought to be initiated by factors termed initiating factors (4,6,19), but this viewpoint apparently has fallen into disfavor (8). The known components that constitute this pathway are properdin (P), native C3 and its large fragment C3b, factor B, factor $\overline{\text{D}}$, magnesium ions, the C3b inactivator (C3b INA), and a plasma protein termed β_1H. One viewpoint of the pathway is described in Fearon and Austen (8). In brief, there are two C3 convertases in the pathway: (1) a priming convertase $\overline{\text{C3,Bb}}$ that continuously cleaves native C3 to provide a supply of C3b, and (2) an amplification convertase $\overline{\text{C3b,Bb}}$ that also cleaves C3, thus providing C3b for these convertases. The term amplification is used because of the feedback of C3b to form more of the alternative pathway C3 convertase $\overline{\text{C3b,Bb}}$.

Factor B and C3b (or C3) form a weak complex (C3b,B), and B is activated by $\overline{\text{D}}$, a serine protease, in the presence of magnesium ions. Factor B activation results in the release of a small fragment Ba that has been reported to be chemotactic for PMN leukocytes. The major portion (Bb) remains bound to C3b (or C3) to form $\overline{\text{C3b,Bb}}$. P may bind to C3b in the complex, preventing the rapid decay of this otherwise short-lived enzyme $\overline{\text{C3b,Bb}}$, but P is not required for the reaction to occur. The C3 convertase $\overline{\text{C3b,Bb}}$ is now capable of cleaving C3 to C3a and C3b, resulting in positive feedback. Amino acid analyses of B have identified it as belonging to the family of serine proteases. Thus Figures 1 and 2 show that the major fragment C3b may be derived from the action of the convertases (1) $\overline{\text{C3,Bb}}$, (2) $\overline{\text{C3b,Bb}}$, (3) $\overline{\text{C4b,2a}}$ of the classic pathway, and (4) possibly from the action of tissue and humoral proteases on native C3.

Similar to the classic pathway C3 convertase, the alternative pathway C3 convertase $\overline{\text{C3b,Bb}}$ binds a second molecule of C3b to form $\overline{\text{C3b,Bb,C3b}}$. The latter cleaves C5 to C5a and C5b and thus is termed a C5 convertase. Properdin also stabilizes this convertase. The product C5b then may interact with the terminal components C6 to C9.

The alternative C pathway is regulated by two proteins, the endopeptidase C3b INA and a plasma globulin β_1H. C3b INA also causes the inactivation of either cellbound or free C3b and C4b of the classic pathway. In the case of bound C3b, β_1H controls both the formation and function of $\overline{\text{C3b,Bb}}$ because it competes with factor B and Bb for the C3b portion of the convertase (20,21). Thus β_1H may block the formation of $\overline{\text{C3b,B}}$ and also cause B or Bb to dissociate from the complex, allowing the C3b INA to cleave C3b to an inactive protein designated C3b′. The latter species has its alpha chain cleaved;

because of this it no longer is able to react in the immune-adherence reaction (22). Further degradation of cellbound C3b′ occurs following the action of proteases such as trypsin, leaving only the C3d portion on a cell membrane (Fig. 2).

The binding affinity of β_1H or factor B for C3b on a membrane is controlled by surface-sialic acid as well as by heparin. This control mechanism is discussed in Fearon and Austen (8). A description of the peptide chains of some of the C proteins and their sites of enzymic hydrolysis are found in Fothergill and Anderson (5).

Another regulatory protein of the alternative pathway C3 convertase $\overline{\text{C3b,Bb}}$, called the C3 nephritic factor, has been described (23,24). The factor is found in some patients with membranoproliferative glomerulonephritis as well as in patients with partial lipodystrophy. It is an autoantibody of the IgG class that binds specifically to $\overline{\text{C3b,Bb}}$. The latter is stabilized by the C3 nephritic factor and results in the depletion of C3 levels in these patients, but the levels of C1, C4, and C2 of the classic pathway are within the normal range. The stabilized convertase is resistant to the action of β_1H (25).

It now is apparent that activation of the C system via the classic or alternative pathways generates a variety of biologically active factors. In inflammed areas, the chemotactic factors attract PMN leukocytes and other inflammatory cells from the circulation. These cells discharge potent enzymes and other factors from lysosomal granules that cause tissue injury and destruction, leading or contributing to the acute and chronic inflammation characteristic of many patients with connective tissue diseases.

CLINICAL APPLICATION OF COMPLEMENT ASSAYS

The measurement of total hemolytic C and of individual C proteins and cleavage products in biologic fluids may provide critical data for the diagnosis and management of diseases with immunologic mechanisms, such as the connective tissue disorders. Thus decreased levels of total C and specific C components have been observed consistently in pathologic sera and other biologic fluids. Immunofluorescent studies of biopsy and autopsy samples have shown deposits of C components, sometimes together with immunoglobulins, on membranes at sites of tissue injury. For example, membrane deposition of immunoglobulins and C in involved skin areas occurs in at least 90%

of patients with SLE. In addition, hypocomplementemia frequently is a clue to the presence of active nephritis in SLE, poststreptococcal infections, congenital nephrosis, and other types of nephritides.

In some immunologically mediated diseases, C quantification may be used not only to confirm the diagnosis but also for follow-up of patients during periods of remission. A decreased serum C level precedes, occasionally by weeks, the clinical signs of exacerbation. Tests for C components may be used in combination with other laboratory tests, such as investigation of anti-DNA antibodies and RF, as a guide for adjusting the treatment of these patients. Whole C levels and quantification of serum C3 and C4 levels by functional or immunochemical assays often will give useful information regarding the immune status of the patient with a connective tissue disease.

COMPLEMENT DEFICIENCY STATES AND DISEASE: ASSOCIATION WITH IMMUNOGENETICS

The availability of reagents for testing all the serum C components and the C inhibitors and inactivators by functional hemolytic assays and by immunochemical methods with specific antibodies have disclosed a number of C deficiency states in human beings. Studies of these deficiencies in families have provided useful information regarding the role of C and its control proteins in natural defense mechanisms (chemotaxis, immune adherence, enhanced phagocytosis, leukocyte mobilization), in the inflammatory process, and in diseases where antigen-antibody complexes contribute to tissue destruction. In addition, it has been shown that certain proteins associated with the C system interact with other biological effector systems, such as kallikreins, enzymes of the clotting cascade, and proteolytic enzymes such as plasmin.

Reports in the literature have described genetic deficiencies for C1r, C1s, C2, C3, C4, C5 (both protein and functional abnormalities), C6, C7, C8, C1 inhibitor (both protein and functional abnormalities), and the C3b inactivator. Other deficiencies have been reported (e.g., C1q), but their causes have not been determined. To date, abnormalities have not been described for factors B and $\overline{D}$, properdin, C9, a C1q inhibitor, anaphylatoxin inactivator, β_1H, and some inhibitors of the terminal C components (6). It is stressed that not all the individuals with deficiencies have unusual clinical problems; in fact, some of them respond normally.

An important recent development from studies of families with C deficiencies is the recognition of a linkage between the genes that control the structure or regulation of specific C components and the genes of the major histocompatibility complex (MHC) (26–31). The C2, C4, C6, and C8 deficiencies as well as the polymorphism of factor B appear to be controlled by genetic determinants that are closely linked to the human MHC (the HLA region). A very small area of human chromosome 6 is associated with at least some of the structural or regulatory C genes as well as with the immune-function gene complex. Thus genes determining the C component deficiencies could be linked to those predisposing to diseases such as the connective tissue

TABLE 1
Genetic Abnormalities
of the Human Complement System and Associated Diseases

Protein deficiency or dysfunction	Clinical disease	Description
C1 esterase inhibitor	Yes	Hereditary angioedema; systemic lupus erythematosus (SLE)-like disease; discoid lupus erythematosus
C1q[a]	Yes	Immunodeficiency
C1q[a]	Yes	Repeated infections
C1r	Yes	SLE and glomerulonephritis
C1s	Yes	SLE and glomerulonephritis
C4	Variable	SLE-like syndrome
C2	Variable	SLE and glomerulonephritis
C3	Yes	Repeated infections
C3b inactivator	Yes	Repeated infections
C5 (functional defect)	Yes	Repeated infections, Leiner's syndrome
C5 (protein defect)	Yes	SLE-like syndrome; frequent bacterial infections
C6	Yes	Repeated infections; mild Raynaud's phenomenon
C7	Variable	Raynaud's phenomenon; no unusual infections
C8	Yes	Recurrent *Neisseria* infections

[a] Genetic association unclear.

disorders, although the existence of such genes has not been established.

The genetic abnormalities of the complement system in human beings and some of the associated clinical problems are listed in Table 1. These are discussed sequentially in the following sections. A more detailed discussion of these problems is found in Opferkuch, Rother, and Schultz (7).

C1 ESTERASE INHIBITOR

The inherited deficiency of this plasma protein in patients with angioedema was first discovered by Donaldson and Evans in 1963 (32). Without a functional inhibitor, C1 is sporadically activated, resulting in the consumption of its substrates C4 and C2 in plasma. It appears that the angioedema is caused by a kinin (C-kinin) derived from C2. With excessive levels of $C\overline{1s}$, C2 is cleaved, plasmin reacts with one of the cleavage products of C2 (Fig. 1), and the kinin is released. The precise mechanism is unclear, but with the release of the kinin, the edema is manifested because of the localized release of vasoactive factors (6,33). The disease is transmitted as an autosomal dominant characteristic.

A few of the patients with this disease have had a SLE-like syndrome or discoid lupus, but the connection between them, if any, is unknown.

Clinically, angioedema is characterized by episodic attacks of acute, circumscribed, and transient edema of the skin, commonly involving part of the face and the extremities. The edema cannot be pitted, it does not itch, there is no discoloration, and it usually disappears in 2 or 3 days. Other features include involvement of the gastrointestinal tract with pain because of the accumulation of edema fluid; occasionally the disease is life threatening because of swelling of the glottis and larynx. Clinical aspects of the disease are discussed in detail elsewhere (34).

Immunochemical and functional assays have shown that most of the patients with angioedema (85%) have low levels of the inhibitor protein, whereas the remainder (15%) have normal or high concentrations, but with little or no function (35). The functional tests for the C1 inhibitor defect measure the patient's serum lack of inhibition of activated C1 for various substrates. For example, Levy and Lepow

(36) developed an assay that measures the action of serum C$\bar{1}$ on the synthetic compound N-acetyl-L-tryosine-ethyl ester. With normal serum the hydrolysis of the ester by C$\bar{1}$ is inhibited by the C1 inhibitor under the conditions of the assay. With serum from a patient with angioedema, C$\bar{1}$ is only partly inhibited or not at all. The same principle is applicable to a hemolytic assay that measures the degree of inhibition of a defined number of units of C$\bar{1}$. The serum C$\bar{1}$ mixture is incubated with sheep erythrocytes sensitized with antibody to which C4b is bound (EAC4 cells). Then C2 and the remaining C components are added and the oxyhemoglobin level is read spectrophotometrically (37).

Since both C4 and C2 are the natural substrates of C$\bar{1}$, the levels of these proteins are low in the serum of individuals with a dysfunctional C1 inhibitor during symptomatic periods. In asymptomatic periods, C2 titers are usually normal, but C4 levels are consistently depressed. C3 and other late-acting components are within the normal range. Thus it is informative to measure C4 by either immunochemical or functional hemolytic methods.

In addition to its function as a modulator of C$\bar{1}$, the C1 inhibitor has a broad spectrum of inhibitory properties: these include inhibition of activated Hageman factor (Factor XII), activated Factor XI (plasma thromboplastin antecedent), a kallikrein that releases bradykinin from plasma kininogen, plasmin, and some other proteases. In cases where the C1 inhibitor is absent or dysfunctional, each or all of these effector proteins may contribute to the pathogenesis of the disease. It is known, for example, that both plasmin and kallikrein can activate C1 directly, leading to consumption of C4 and C2 and the release of the C kinin.

C1q

A partial or complete deficiency of C1q (a subcomponent of the first component of C, Fig. 1) levels has been described in some but not all patients with hypogammaglobulinemia and severe combined immunodeficiency disease (38). In some patients with this deficiency, the problems associated with lymphopenia, hypogammaglobulinemia, and infection are so severe that the effects of the C1q deficiency cannot be studied. Although the levels of C1q are low, the levels of C1s are relatively normal, suggesting that C1s and C1q are not linked (39).

A young boy was described with undetectable levels of C1q protein and C1q activity but with normal levels of C1r, C1s, and the other C components (40). The patient had continuous problems with severe infections that could not be explained by low levels of immunoglobulins because the levels of IgG, IgA, and IgM were within the normal range. The cause of this anomaly was not clear.

C1r, C1s

There are a few examples of C1r deficiency associated with a slight depression of C1s and elevated levels of C4 (7). These patients have had SLE and glomerulonephritis of varying severity, but the association of the deficiency, if any, with the disease is obscure. The C1r deficiency is acquired by an autosomal recessive inheritance, whereas at least one family with C1s deficiency is caused by an absence of an autosomal dominant allele.

In studies of the immune adherence and bactericidal activities of the patients' sera deficient in C1r, both these functions were impaired with erythrocytes sensitized with antibody and *Escherichia coli*, respectively.

C4

A few cases of a homozygous deficiency of C4 have been reported; all have had clinical SLE (29,41). In one family study, a 7-year-old boy had no detectable C4 by either immunochemical or functional assays (29). The C abnormality was transmitted as an autosomal recessive trait. Many members of the family were heterozygotes. HLA typing of the child and members of his family showed linkage between the C4-dependent gene and the genes for the major histocompatibility complex.

C2

More cases of C2 deficiency have been studied than of any of the other C component abnormalities (7). Initially, a few healthy persons were discovered with the deficiency, but other cases have been reported with anaphylactoid purpura, SLE, polymyositis, Hodgkin's disease, chronic lymphocytic leukemia, renal diseases, and various connective tissue disorders. As is the case with the other deficiencies of the classic C proteins, it is not clear whether a connection exists between the defect and the susceptibility to the disease. These cases also show that in spite of the deficiencies in C2, or whether the defect is heterozygous or homozygous, a normal, healthy life is possible (42). C2 deficiency also emphasizes the importance of the alternative C pathway in host defense against microbial agents. Low levels of C2 may be transmitted as an autosomal recessive characteristic. Most of the C2-deficient homozygous cases have had disorders involving mesenchymal tissues.

C3

A few patients have been described with a severe deficiency of C3, and one has been extensively studied to learn or confirm the importance of C3 in various immunologic reactions (43). Her serum had no appreciable opsonic or chemotactic activity and was deficient in bactericidal and hemolytic C action. She had frequent pyogenic infections, lobar pneumonia, otitis media, meningococcal meningitis, and other problems. The humoral antibody response in the patient to various protein and carbohydrate antigens was normal. Thus the C3 deficiency and the susceptibility to infectious agents correlate with the important biologic functions of C3 (Figs. 2 and 3). However, a case was described by Osofsky et al. (44) with an immunochemical and hemolytic complete deficiency of C3, but the child was quite healthy. It is evident that in some circumstances the individual can compensate for the C3 deficiency, but the mechanism and the factors are unknown. Although a few heterozygous C3 individuals have been reported with C3 concentrations approximately 50% of normal, they have had no unusual problems with infectious agents. The C3 deficiency is inherited as an autosomal codominant trait.

C3b INACTIVATOR

Another patient with a history of severe bacterial infections was discovered to be homozygous deficient for C3b INA (45). The inactivator is an important modulator of the alternative C pathway. In its absence the C proteins are constantly depleted because of spontaneous activation. This case illustrates again the importance of C3 and the alternative C pathway in providing protection against a wide variety of infectious agents.

C5: FUNCTIONAL AND PROTEIN DEFECTS

In Table 1, the C5 abnormalities have been divided empirically into two groups: the first, a C5 protein that is normal in most functions but impaired in the ability to phagocytize yeast particles (46); the second, a total deficiency of C5 (47). Sera from the latter group promoted phagocytosis of yeast particles normally but were severely impaired in the generation of chemotactic activity. C5 deficiency is inherited as an autosomal codominant trait. Some persons in both groups, i.e., with the functional or protein deficiencies, suffered from recurrent infections. Those who were defective in the phagocytosis assays with yeast had a normal C5 as determined by hemolytic and immunochemical criteria. One patient with total C5 deficiency had a lupus-like syndrome and recurrent infections but had a sister with approximately 1% of normal levels of C5 who was healthy. Furthermore, four additional family members had half-normal quantities of C5 and appeared to be healthy. It is apparent that although all these cases are associated with C5, they differ greatly in the nature of the deficiency.

C6

A young female was described with a lack of hemolytic C activity. Detailed experiments showed that she had a complete protein and functional deficiency of C6 (48). The defect appeared to follow classic Mendelian inheritance. The patient had problems with recurrent disseminated gonococcal infections. The family history was negative for infections. A boy was also described with a C6 deficiency who had recurrent meningococcal meningitis (49). The functional properties of other C components were normal.

Although the plasma of rabbits with a C6 deficiency has a retarded rate of blood coagulation, which is corrected by the addition of purified C6, no defect was found in the plasma of a C6-deficient patient (50).

C7

A female patient with Raynaud's phenomenon, sclerodactyly, and telangiectasia was found by Boyer et al. to have a deficiency of C7 (51). No specific inhibitors of C7 were detected in the patient's serum, although a C7-deficient patient with normal health was found by Wellek and Opferkuch to have a C7 inhibitor (52). A puzzling finding with Boyer's patient was the defective phagocytosis of yeast particles and a defect in chemotaxis. Since both C3 and C5 were apparently normal, and since the patient did not have an unusual number of infections, the defective phagocytosis and chemotaxis are difficult to explain. Possibly there is another undetected problem associated with this deficiency or the other complications.

C8

A young female patient was described with a hereditary deficiency of C8 (53). The component was not detectable by functional hemolytic or immunochemical assays. The other C proteins were normal. Addition of purified C8 to her serum restored the deficiency for hemolytic C titrations. The serum lacked bactericidal action against *Neisseria gonorrhoeae,* but purified C8 added to the serum restored this activity. Since most of the known biologic activities of the C system occur prior to the C8 step, the only activity that is missing is cytolysis, which requires C8 and C9. The data indicated that the patient is homozygous for the deficiency. Her children and parents were shown to be heterozygotes with C8 levels approximately 50% of normal.

REFERENCES

1. Schultz DR. The complement system. Monogr Allergy 6:1-131, 1971.
2. Mayer MM. The complement system. Sci Am 229:54-66, 1973.
3. Müller-Eberhard HJ. Complement. Annu Rev Biochem 44:697-724, 1975.
4. Müller-Eberhard HJ. Chemistry and function of the complement system. Hosp Pract 12:33-43, 1977.
5. Fothergill JE, Anderson WHK. A molecular approach to the complement system. In: Horecker BL, Stadtman ER, eds. Current Topics in Cellular Regulation, Vol. 13. New York: Academic Press, p. 259, 1978.
6. Müller-Eberhard HJ. Complement abnormalities in human disease. Hosp Pract 13:65, 1978.
7. Opferkuch W, Rother K, Schultz DR. Clinical Aspects of the Complement System. Stuttgart: G. Thieme, 1978.
8. Fearon DT, Austen KF. The alternative pathway of complement-A system for host resistance to microbial infection. N Engl J Med 303:259-263, 1980.
9. Schultz DR. Complement in host defense. Scand J Infect Dis (Suppl) 24:22-29, 1980.

10. Bokish VA, Müller-Eberhard HJ, Cochrane CG. Anaphylatoxin inactivator of human plasma: its isolation and characterization as a carboxypeptidase. J Clin Invest 49:2427-2436, 1970.
11. Till G, Ward PA. Two distinct chemotactic factor inactivators in human serum. J Immunol 114:843-847, 1975.
12. Loos M, Bitter-Suermann D, Dierich M. Interaction of the first (C1), the second (C2), and the fourth (C4) components of complement with different preparations of bacterial lipopolysaccharides and with lipid A. J Immunol 112:935-940, 1974.
13. Cooper NR. Activation of the complement system. Top Mol Immunol 2:155-183, 1973.
14. Loos M, Wellek B, Thesen R, Opferkuch W. Antibody-independent interaction of the first component of complement with gram-negative bacteria. Infect Immun 22:5-9, 1978.
15. Schultz DR, Loos M, Bub F, Arnold PI. Differentiation of hemolytically active fluid-phase and cell-bound human $C1_q$ by an ant venom-derived polysaccharide. J Immunol 124:1251-1257, 1980.
16. Burnet M. Auto-immunity and Auto-immune Disease. Philadelphia: Davis, 1972.
17. Ziff M. Autoimmune processes in rheumatoid arthritis. Prog Immunol 11:37, 1974.
18. Pillemer L, Blum L, Lepow IH, et al. The properdin system and immunity: I. Demonstration and isolation of a new serum protein, properdin, and its role in immune phenomena. Science 120:279-285, 1954.
19. Medicus RG, Schreiber RD, Götze O, et al. A molecular concept of the properdin pathway. Proc Natl Acad Sci 73:612-616, 1976.
20. Whaley K, Ruddy S. Modulation of the alternative complement pathway by β_1H globulin. J Exp Med 144:1147-1163, 1976.
21. Weiler JM, Daha MR, Austen KF, Fearon DT. Control of the amplification convertase of complement by the plasma protein β_1H. Proc Natl Acad Sci 73:3268-3272, 1976.
22. Law SK, Fearon DT, Levine RP. Action of the C3b-inactivator on cell-bound C3b. J Immunol 122:759-765, 1979.
23. Spitzer RE, Vallota EH, Forristal J, et al. Serum C3 lytic system in patients with glomerulonephritis. Science 164:436-437, 1969.
24. Schreiber RD, Götze O, Müller-Eberhard HJ. Alternative pathway of complement: demonstration and characterization of initiating factor and its properdin-independent function. J Exp Med 144:1062-1075, 1976.
25. Daha MR, Austen KF, Fearon DT. Heterogeneity, polypeptide chain composition and antigenic reactivity of C3 nephritic factor. J Immunol 120:1389-1394, 1978.
26. Day NK, L'Esperance P, Good RA, et al. Hereditary C2 deficiency. Genetic studies and association with the HLA system. J Exp Med 141:1464-1469, 1975.
27. Gibson DJ, Glass D, Carpenter CB, et al. Hereditary C2 deficiency: diagnosis and HLA gene complex associations. J Immunol 116:1065-1070, 1976.

28. Raum D, Glass D, Carpenter CB, et al. The chromosomal order of genes controlling the major histocompatibility complex, properdin factor B, and deficiency of the second component of complement. J Clin Invest 58:1240-1248, 1976.
29. Ochs HD, Rosenfeld SI, Thomas ED, et al. Linkage between the gene (or genes) controlling synthesis of the fourth component of complement and the major histocompatibility complex. N Engl J Med 296:470-475, 1977.
30. Raum D, Glass D, Carpenter CB, et al. C6 deficiency-HLA association. Fed Proc 35:655, 1976.
31. Merritt AD, Petersen BH, Biegel AA, et al. Chromosome 6: Linkage of the eighth component of complement (C8) to the histocompatibility region (HLA): human gene mapping 3. Balt Conf Birth Defects 7:331-334, 1976.
32. Donaldson VH, Evans RR. A biochemical abnormality in hereditary angioneurotic edema: absence of serum inhibitor of C1-esterase. Am J Med 35:37-44, 1963.
33. Donaldson VH, Ratnoff OD, Klemperer MR, et al. Studies on a peptide from hereditary angioneurotic edema plasma with permeability factor and kinin activity. J Immunol 101:818, 1968.
34. Austen KF. Inborn and acquired abnormalities of the complement system of man. Johns Hopkins Med J 128:57-74, 1971.
35. Rosen FS, Charache P, Pensky J, et al. Hereditary angioneurotic edema: two genetic variants. Science 148:957-958, 1965.
36. Levy LR, Lepow IH. Assay and properties of a serum inhibitor of C1 esterase. Proc Soc Exp Biol Med 101:608-614, 1959.
37. Ruddy S, Gigli I, Sheffer AL, et al. The laboratory diagnosis of hereditary angioedema. In: Rose B, Richter M, Sehon A, eds. Allergology. Proceedings of the Sixth Congress of the International Association of Allergology. Amsterdam: Excerpta Medica, p. 351, 1968.
38. Gewurz H, Pickering RJ, Christian CL, et al. Decreased $C1_q$ protein concentration and agglutinating activity in agammaglobulinemia syndromes: an inborn error reflected in the complement system. Clin Exp Immunol 3:437-445, 1968.
39. Stroud RM, Nagaki K, Pickering RJ, et al. Subunits of the first complement component in immunologic deficiency syndromes: independence of C1s and C1q. Clin Exp Immunol 7:133-137, 1970.
40. Berkel AI, Sanal O, Thesen R, Loos M. A case of selective C1q deficiency. Turkish J Pediatr 19:101, 1977.
41. Hauptman G, Grosshans E, Heid E, et al. Lupus erythematosus aigu avec deficit complet de la fraction C4 du complement. Nouv Presse Med 3:881-882, 1974.
42. Glass D, Raum D, Gibson D, et al. Inherited deficiency of the second component of complement: rheumatic disease associations. J Clin Invest 58:853-861, 1976.
43. Alper CA, Colten HR, Gear JSS, et al. Homozygous human C3 deficiency: the role of C3 in antibody production, $C\bar{1}s$-induced vasoperme-

ability, and cobra venom-induced passive hemolysis. J Clin Invest 57:222-229, 1976.

44. Osofsky S, Thompson BH, Lint TF, Gewurz H. Hereditary deficiency of the third component of complement in a child with fever, skin rash, and arthralgias: response to transfusion of whole blood. J Pediatr 90:180-186, 1977.
45. Alper CH, Rosen FS. The role of complement in vivo as revealed by genetic defects. In: Brent L, Holborrow J, eds. Progress in Immunology II, Vol. 1. Amsterdam: North-Holland, p. 201, 1974.
46. Miller ME, Nilsson UR. A familial deficiency of the phagocytosis enhancing activity of serum related to a dysfunction of the fifth component of complement (C5). N Engl J Med 282:354-358, 1970.
47. Rosenfeld SI, Leddy JP. Hereditary deficiency of fifth component of complement (C5) in man. J Clin Invest 57:1635-1643, 1976.
48. Leddy JP, Frank MM, Gather T, et al. Hereditary deficiency of the sixth component of complement in man: I. Immunochemical, biologic, and family studies. J Clin Invest 53:544-553, 1974.
49. Gewurz A, Lim D, Ghaze M, et al. Absence of C6 with recurrent meningococcal meningitis. Clin Res 23:532A, 1975.
50. Heusinkveld RS, Leddy JP, Klemperer MR, et al. Hereditary deficiency of the sixth component of complement in man: II. Studies of hemostasis. J Clin Invest 53:554-558, 1974.
51. Boyer JT, Gall EP, Norman ME, et al. Hereditary deficiency of the seventh component of complement. J Clin Invest 56:905-913, 1975.
52. Wellek B, Opferkuch W. A naturally occurring C7 inactivator in a case of C7 deficiency in man and in normal human serum. Fed Proc 33:648, 1974.
53. Petersen BH, Graham JA, Brooks GF. Human deficiency of the eighth component of complement: the requirement of C8 for serum Neisseria gonorrhoeae bactericidal activity. J Clin Invest 57:283-290, 1976.

SEROLOGY

DUANE R. SCHULTZ, Ph.D.

RHEUMATOID FACTORS

Rheumatoid factors (RF) are associated with autoimmune processes and are defined as anti-gamma globulin antibodies with major specificity directed toward the Fc fragment on autologous, isologous, and heterologous subclasses of IgG (1,2). The anti-gamma globulin is usually of the IgM and IgG classes, but IgA and secretory IgA (3) as well as 7S IgM (4) have also been reported. IgD and IgE are not important in rheumatoid arthritis (RA).

RF is detected in the patient's serum by using IgG (usually human or rabbit) chemically coupled to sheep erythrocytes, polyaminopolystyrene particles, or bentonite. A positive test is indicated by an agglutination or flocculation reaction. Immunofluorescent staining of tissue sections (using fluorescein-labeled, aggregated, denatured IgG) is also a useful technique for demonstrating RF. The IgM-RF has a low association constant for IgG and thus is easily dissociated at physiologic pH values. Occasionally, RF-IgG complexes cryoprecipitate at temperatures below 37° C.

RF-IgG complexes fix complement. This reaction probably has phlogistic importance in the pathogenesis of RA. For example, chemotaxis of polymorphonuclear leukocytes occurs following the interaction of RF, IgG, and fresh serum as a source of complement. The chemotactic factors may be derived from cleaved complement proteins. RF may alter the size or solubility of immune complexes, allowing increased phagocytosis by leukocytes. In addition, RF enhances complement-mediated lysis of erythrocytes sensitized with small quantities of IgG antibody(5).

Severe cases of RA with extraarticular symptoms usually have a high titer of RF, intracytoplasmic inclusions of denatured immunoglobulin, and a decreased complement titer in synovial fluid. Both immunoglobulins and complement components are synthesized in areas that are commonly inflamed in arthritis, such as knee joints. The evidence that RF-IgG complexes activate various effector systems such as complement demonstrates their important role in the inflammatory process. Seropositive patients followed for years usually have had a more severe disease than those who are seronegative. Small quantities of RF also are produced in some seronegative patients; IgM has been found in synovial fluid polymorphonuclear leukocytes. In other connective tissue diseases such as systemic lupus erythematosus (SLE), approximately 15% of cases have a positive RF.

Therefore, the current opinion is that RF, in complexes with IgG, plays an important role as an activator of effector systems such as complement. These systems may initiate the inflammatory process in synovial tissues or in the local blood circulation because of the production of chemotactic factors, causing local aggregation of polymorphonuclear leukocytes. Increased phagocytosis by these cells as well as by cells in the synovial lining layer causes the release from their lysosomal granules of potent hydrolytic enzymes. These factors are responsible for much of the tissue damage in inflammation.

ANTINUCLEAR ANTIBODIES (ANA)

Antigen-antibody complexes either directly or indirectly cause much of the tissue damage in connective tissue diseases (6). Although the serologic picture of patients with these diseases is by no means uniform, most have antibodies to autoantigens. In SLE, the antibodies characteristically react with a wide variety of cellular and humoral antigens. These include single- and double-stranded (native) DNA, double-stranded RNA, DNA histone, nucleoprotein, histone, extractable nuclear antigen, and a saline-soluble nuclear factor (Sm) (6,7). There are also serum antibodies to coagulation factors, red and white blood cell components, cardiolipin, and platelets. The antibodies are found in patients in all four IgG subclasses in a distribution similar to that of normal human serum. Since IgG1 and IgG3 subclasses fix complement more efficiently than does IgG2 (IgG4 does not fix complement), they are usually associated with cases having active lupus nephritis and low serum complement (8). Antinuclear antibodies may also be of the IgM and IgA classes.

Positive tests for ANA have been demonstrated in most patients treated with hydralazine and procainamide (9). Although currently hydralazine is infrequently prescribed, procainamide is widely used for the control of cardiac irregularity. There is no evidence of kidney involvement, and other symptoms usually disappear in a few weeks after discontinuing the drug.

It is informative not only to test for the presence and quantity of the ANA, but also to identify the specificities of the ANA in patient's sera (10). If possible, the tests should be repeated within a reasonable period of time (weeks) in order to aid or confirm the diagnosis, management, and treatment of the disease.

In reference to antibodies to DNA, at least three major classes have been described in various connective tissue disorders: (1) antibodies to double-stranded (native) DNA (DS-DNA), (2) antibodies that react with both DS-DNA and single-stranded DNA (SS-DNA), and (3) antibodies that react solely with SS-DNA. It is important to distinguish between these classes because of false-positive reactions. A serum with a high titer of antibodies to DS-DNA often is associated with systemic lupus erythematosus (SLE) and nephritis. Antibodies to SS-DNA usually have no specificity for either SLE or nephritis and are frequently found in all connective tissue diseases. Therefore, the DNA preparations used as antigen in the immunological assays must be 100% DS-DNA; otherwise, with contaminating SS-DNA, misleading results may be obtained. For example, one of the assays commonly used where this has been a problem is the sensitive radioimmunoassay: the DNA is radiolabeled, then reacted with the patient's serum which may contain antibodies to both DS- and SS-DNA. Another technical problem with the radioimmunoassay for DS-DNA antibodies is the binding of DNA to factors other than antibody, giving the impression of a specific antigen-antibody reaction.

Antibodies to SM antigen, a nonhistone acidic nuclear protein, are detected by a number of different assays (see following). Approximately 30% of the sera from patients with SLE contain these antibodies. Since it is unusual to find these antibodies in other connective tissue disorders, it is desirable to test for them.

Considerable evidence exists that immune complexes comprised of autoantigens and their specific antibodies are formed in patients with

SLE during periods of disease activity or progressive renal lesions. For example, there is a good correlation between the presence of DS-DNA-anti-DNA antibody complexes and nephritis (7). In addition, antibodies may be bound to the basement membrane of skin in as many as 90% of patients in SLE (7,11). The immune complexes formed in the presence of excess antibody most frequently are insoluble and may be rapidly eliminated by reticuloendothelial cells. Complexes formed at equivalence or in the presence of slight antigen excess are usually soluble and may be deposited in renal glomeruli, the skin, the synovial membrane of joints, and walls of small vessels. In the renal glomerulus, immune complexes may be deposited on the epithelial side of the basement membrane, in skin venules, in the capillary loops of the dermal papillae (particularly around basement membranes), and in arteries, where the elastic lamina is the main site of deposition. These complexes have a high affinity for complement, which is activated. The products of this activation as well as from other effector systems, such as kallikreins and plasmin, lead to an accumulation of polymorphonuclear leukocytes. Lysis of these cells results in the release of potent lysosomal proteases (7) that cause tissue destruction.

There are several direct and indirect tests to detect ANA (10). These include the LE-cell test, direct and indirect immunofluorescence, double diffusion in gel, antiglobulin consumption, complement fixation, counterimmunoelectrophoresis, hemagglutination, and radioimmunoassay. The indirect immunofluorescent assay is commonly used to screen sera; a negative result will practically eliminate the possibility of SLE unless the patient is on immunosuppressive or steroid therapy. Nevertheless, immunofluorescent assays do not detect all ANA because negative reactions have been reported from patients with polymyositis, scleroderma, and Sjögren's syndrome, although their sera showed precipitating antibodies by other immunological assays. DNA of any origin will serve as antigen in these tests, but usually cells with large nuclei, such as mouse fibroblasts, are selected. A positive test appears as one of the following morphologic types of nuclear fluorescence: homogeneous (diffuse), membranous (outlined, shaggy), speckled, or nucleolar.

The homogeneous type of fluorescent staining, the most common in discoid lupus and SLE, is caused by anti-DNA and antinucleoprotein antibody (11). The next most frequent type, speckled fluorescence, is caused by antibody to the Sm antigen. The nucleolar pattern, caused by ANA reacting with RNA, is infrequently seen in SLE. The membranous type is indicative of high-titer DNA antibodies; usually, patients with this pattern are seriously ill. Occasionally there is more than one pattern. These are more clearly delineated by serially diluting the patient's serum. A low-titer antibody will be eliminated by dilution, allowing a second, high-titer antibody to react in the fluorescent staining test.

HISTOCOMPATIBILITY ANTIGENS (HLA)

Investigations of whether tissue or organ allografts would be subject to immunologic rejection in human beings and other vertebrates eventually led to the discovery of the leukocyte system of isoantigens, including the human leukocyte antigen, or locus A (HLA) system. This genetic regulatory region is termed the major histocompatibility complex, or MHC (Table 1). Tests for this complex attempt to identify the tissue antigen products of the MHC of different people and to match donor-recipient pairs for organ or tissue transplantation on the basis of their possessing some of these antigens in common. Four HLA antigens were discovered on autosome number 6 in Caucasians. It is thought that they are transmitted by two related loci on each of a pair of chromosomes. These closely linked loci are inherited as a unit, each of which is termed a haplotype (12). Alleles for loci A, B, and C are defined serologically (SD) with specific antisera. The D locus antigens are lymphocyte defined (LD). A loose linkage occurs between MHC and other chromosomal markers such as phosphoglucomutase 3, glyoxyalase, and urinary pepsinogen 5. More closely linked are the loci controlling certain complement components such as C2 and C4 (see the first chapter).

Several studies have attempted to find an association between HLA and specific diseases (13–17). It now is thought that HLA-linked, specific immune response (Ir) genes are important hereditary factors that predispose the individual to states of susceptibility or resistance to autoimmune, malignant, and infectious diseases.

The antigens of the HLA system are detected by serologic methods and are identified by increases in antigen frequency in patients with specific diseases. Thus the lymphocytes of patients and controls are tested in lymphocyte toxicity trials against a panel of different, spe-

TABLE 1
Some Commonly Used Terms and Their Definitions for the Genetics of Immune Disorders of Human Beings

Abbreviation or term	Definition
MHC	*Major histocompatibility complex.* Cluster of linked genes that controls the major histocompatibility antigens expressed on the surface of nucleated cells.
HLA	The MHC of human beings: the system of antigens first detected on human leukocytes. (Human leukocyte antigen, or human leukocyte locus A.)
Autosome	A chromosome that is not a sex chromosome.
Phenotype	The outward visible expression of a trait that is inherited.
Genotype	The genetic composition of the individual.
Allele	One of an array of possible mutational forms of a given gene.
Linkage	Greater association in inheritance of two or more nonallelic genes than is to be expected from independent assortment. Genes are linked because they are found on the same chromosome.
Locus (pl., loci)	Position that a gene occupies and codes for a trait in a chromosome.
SD	*Serologically defined* histocompatibility antigens determined by loci A, B, and C of the MHC.
LD	*Lymphocyte defined* histocompatibility antigens. Designated by locus D of the MHC, they determine the ability of lymphocytes from one person to stimulate those of a second person in mixed lymphocyte culture. Previously called MLC (mixed lymphocyte culture) or MLR (mixed lymphocyte reactivity).
Ir	*Immune response* genes: loci within the MHC that control whether an immune response occurs to a specific antigen and its magnitude.
Haplotype	Entire genetic complex inherited from one parent in terms of MHC loci A to D.

cific typing sera (18). The results of these tests indicate an association between genes in the HLA region that control the immune response of an individual to a certain disease.

Within the past few years, one of the specifically identifiable histocompatibility antigens, the HLA-B27, has been found in a high proportion of patients (72 of 75) with ankylosing spondylitis and in 32 of 60 first-degree relatives (13). The observations have been extended to include its presence in 47 of 63 patients with Reiter's disease and in 26 of 29 patients with psoriatic arthritis. Also, HLA-B27 was found in 29 of 33 patients with acute anterior uveitis with associated diseases reporting to an eye department in England. It was present in 13 of 18 patients with ulcerative colitis and spondylitis, in 4 of 5 patients with Crohn's disease and spondylitis, and in 14 of 15 patients with arthritis following *Salmonella* infection. In Finland, HLA-B27 has been reported in 43 of 49 patients with *Yersinia* arthritis. Therefore, HLA-B27 is associated with a large number of inflammatory disorders. The possibility of a common mechanism must be considered.

There are many important questions concerning the relationship of histocompatibility antigens and susceptibility or resistance to various diseases (19). For example, are these antigens merely genetic markers, or do they contribute to the development of the disease? The ultimate answer may be the the most significant outcome of these investigations. However, these studies undoubtedly justify the effect involved in maintaining laboratory tests to aid in diagnosis in practical rheumatology and other clinical divisions and departments.

REFERENCES

1. Munthe E, Natvig JB. Immunoglobulin classes, subclasses, and complexes of IgG rheumatoid factor in rheumatoid plasma cells. Clin Exp Immunol 12:55–70, 1972.
2. Stage DE, Mannik M. Rheumatoid factors in rheumatoid arthritis. Bull Rheum Dis 23:720–725, 1972.
3. Abraham GN, Clark RA, Vaughan JH. Characterization of an IgA rheumatoid factor. Binding properties and reactivity with the subclasses of human γG globulin. Immunochemistry 9:301–315, 1972.
4. Stage DE, Mannik M. 7S γM globulins and 7S γM rheumatoid factor in patients with rheumatoid arthritis. Arthritis Rheum 12:699, 1969.
5. Schmid FR, Roitt IM, Rocha MJ. Complement fixation by a two-component antibody system: immunoglobulin G and immunoglobulin M antiglobulin (rheumatoid factor). J Exp Med 132:673–693, 1970.
6. Tuffanelli D. Lupus erythematosus. Arch Dermatol 106:553–556, 1972.
7. Reichlin M, Mattioli M. Antigens and antibodies characteristic of systemic lupus erythematosus. Bull Rheum Dis 24:756–760, 1973.
8. Schur PH, Monroe M, Rothfield N. The γG subclass of antinuclear and antinucleic acid antibodies. Arthritis Rheum 15:174–182, 1972.
9. Condemi JJ, Blomgren SE, Vaughan JH. The procainamide-induced lupus syndrome. Bull Rheum Dis 20:604–607, 1970.

10. Notman DD, Kurata N, and Tan EM. Profiles of antinuclear antibodies in systemic rheumatic disease. Ann Intern Med 83:464–469, 1975.
11. Kay DM, Tuffanelli DL. Immunofluorescent techniques in clinical diagnosis of cutaneous disease. Ann Intern Med 71:753-762, 1969.
12. WHO-IUIS Terminology Committee. Nomenclature for factors of the HLA system-1977. Transplantation 25:272-275, 1978.
13. Brewerton DA, James DCO. The histocompatibility antigen (HL/AB27) and disease. Semin Arthritis Rheum 4:191-207, 1975.
14. McDevitt HO, Bodmer WF. HL-A, immune-response genes, and disease. Lancet 1:1269-1275, 1974.
15. Brewerton DA, Hart FD, Nicholls A, et al. Ankylosing spondylitis and HL-A 27. Lancet 1:904, 1974.
16. Amor B, Feldmann JL, Delbarre F, et al. HL-A antigen W27: a genetic link between ankylosing spondylitis and Reiter's syndrome? N Engl J Med 290:572, 1974.
17. Dausset J, Svejgaard A. HLA and Disease. Copenhagen: Munksgaard, 1977.
18. Terasaki PI, McClelland JD. Microdroplet assay of human serum cytotoxins. Nature 204:998-1000, 1964.
19. Woodrow JC. Histocompatibility antigens. Semin Arthritis Rheum 6:257-276, 1977.

MEDIATORS OF THE INFLAMMATORY PROCESS

DUANE R. SCHULTZ, Ph.D.

FACTOR XII (HAGEMAN FACTOR) ACTIVATED SYSTEMS

Several developments regarding the functions of blood clotting Factor XII (Hageman factor) in the inflammatory response have led to the overall reaction scheme shown in Figure 1 (1–5). The scheme emphasizes the interrelationships of the clotting, kinin, fibrinolytic, and complement pathways. The last named system was discussed in the first chapter.

Factor XII is activated by a number of substances such as glass, kaolin, celite, collagen, and vascular basement membranes or other surfaces and factors with dense negative charges (6). The reaction is enhanced further by high molecular weight kininogen. Activated Factor XII (XIIa) initiates three biologically important pathways: the fibrinolytic, kinin, and intrinsic blood clotting systems. In the absence of Factor XII, the first steps of kinin production and of intrinsic coagulation are not accomplished. These pathways have several inhibitors in common, such as the C1 inhibitor, α_2-macroglobulin, α_1-antitrypsin, and α_2-antithrombin. Each inhibitor acts as a modulator of the various enzyme-substrate interactions (1,7). Plasmin, the final product of the fibrinolytic cascade, kallikrein in the kinin system, and Factor XI in the intrinsic clotting pathway are all capable of activating Factor XII, resulting in a positive feedback mechanism (3,8). In addition, plasmin can activate C1 and C3 in the complement system and kallikrein can activate C1. Both reactions with C1 are inhibited by the C1 inhibitor (7).

Several forms of Factor XII have been reported. One of them (MW 90,000) is dissociated after reduction or cleavage to three subunit

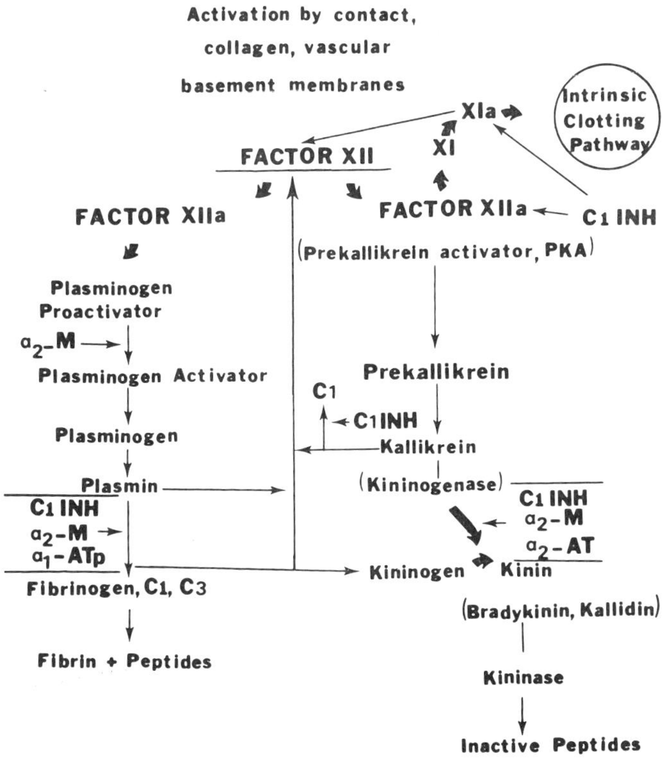

FIGURE 1

Summary of blood clotting Factor XII (Hageman factor) activated systems. (C1 INH = C1 inhibitor; α_2-M = α_2 macroglobulin; α_2-AT = α_2-antithrombin; α_1-ATp = α_1-antitrypsin.)

fragments having an electrophoretic mobility similar to that of prealbumin, with a MW of 30,000 each (8,9). The fragments, referred to as prealbumin activator β-XIIa, or prekallikrein activator (PKA), have most of the activities of the parent molecule but have lost a small amount of the clot-promoting activity (8). These fragments were implicated as the cause of hypotension in surgical cases receiving plasma protein fraction (mostly albumin) for volume expansion (5). Presumably this was caused by the production of bradykinin in the patients. Although neither Factor XII nor XIIa is susceptible to diisopropylfluorophosphate, the subunits are inactivated by this compound.

Factor XIIa has at least three substrates in plasma: prekallikrein

(Fletcher factor), Factor XI (plasma thromboplastin antecedent or PTA), and the plasminogen proactivator (9,10). In addition, these three substrates are activated by PKA. The C1 inhibitor inhibits PKA, Factor XIIa, and Factor XIa. Evidence indicates that Factor XIa is also inhibited by antithrombin III (11) and by α_1-antitrypsin (12). Plasmin, kallikrein, pepsin, trypsin, proteases in snake venoms, and bacterial products can act as kininogenases to produce a kinin from kininogen (Fitzgerald, Reid, Flaujeac, Williams factor). The action of kallikrein produces the nonapeptide bradykinin, and tissue pancreatic kallikrein produces the decapeptide lysyl-bradykinin (called kallidin) (13,14). The latter kinin is a straight-chain polypeptide that resembles bradykinin in its pharmacologic activity. The α_2-macroglobulin, α_2-antithrombin, and the C1 inhibitor all inhibit kallikrein.

Kininases cleave the C-terminal arginine of kinins to inactivate the peptides (14). The amino acid sequence of two kinins with amino- and carboxyl-terminal ends are as follows:

NH_2-Arg-Pro-Pro-Gly-Phe-Ser-Pro-Phe-Arg-COOH
(bradykinin)

If Lys- is located on the N-terminal end, the kinin is kallidin (decapeptide).

Kallikrein has also been shown to activate C1 and is chemotactic for polymorphonuclear leukocytes (15). Nanogram amounts of the kinins induce the cardinal features of the inflammatory response including pain, vasodilation, enhanced capillary permeability, and chemotaxis. The major effector agent of the kinin system is bradykinin (14).

Thus the plasma kallikrein-kinin system participates in a variety of states where inflammation is a feature, including arthritis, shock, allergies, and burns. A sensitive radioimmunoassay has been developed that measures prekallikrein and kallikrein in various clinical disorders (16).

The final step of part of the enzyme-substrate cascade shown in Figure 1 is the conversion of fibrinogen to fibrin and the release of fibrinopeptides. These factors are important in some coagulation abnormalities and in connective tissue diseases and may be the lethal factor in some types of glomerulonephritis.

The action of the plasma proteinase thrombin on soluble fibrinogen results in the hydrolysis of several small fibrinopeptides designated A, AP, AY, and B (17). First the A and finally the B peptides on each fibrinogen monomer are hydrolyzed from the N-terminal ends. The final result is the formation of fibrin monomers, which aggregate or polymerize to insoluble forms by end-to-end and side-to-side hydrogen bonding. Thrombin-activated Factor XIII is a transamidase that converts H-bond fibrin polymers to more stable, covalently bonded forms. After thrombin-induced clot formation occurs, serum possesses chemotactic activity for peripheral blood leukocytes (18). Furthermore, fibrinopeptide B and not fibrinopeptide A attracts leukocytes, emphasizing the significance of clot formation in the inflammatory process. For example, many patients with glomerulonephritis have excessive fibrin deposition in the glomeruli (19).

The mechanism of action of plasmin is different from that of thrombin: both fibrinogen and fibrin are serially degraded over several intermediates to smaller end products and numerous smaller fragments (20–24). Plasminogen activators derived from endothelial or tissue cells convert plasminogen, which has coprecipitated with fibrin polymers, into plasmin within the interstices of developing fibrin polymer clots (25). During plasmin-induced fibrinolysis, fibrin undergoes serial cleavage into smaller molecules termed X, Y, D, and E. In a presumably analogous in vitro situation with native fibrinogen, the molecular weights of the degradation products are 270,000, 155,000, 90,000, and 30,000 to 50,000, respectively. The degradation derivatives after X are incoagulable by thrombin (26).

PROSTAGLANDINS, THROMBOXANES, AND OTHER PRODUCTS OF FATTY ACID OXIDATION

Prostaglandins (PG) are believed to play an important role as mediators in inflammation. Apparently all cells in the body have the enzymes that are necessary for their synthesis. In particular, PMN-leukocytes in acute inflammation as well as macrophages and lymphocytes in chronic inflammation are able to convert C_{20} polyunsaturated fatty acids to various biologically active products. Biosynthetic pathways leading to the formation of these 20-carbon compounds from the long-chain fatty acids [particularly arachidonic acid, $CH_3(CH_2)_3(CH_2CH{=}CH)_4(CH_2)_3COOH$] have been described (27–32). Thus, when molecular oxygen reacts with the fatty acids in the presence of the enzyme cyclo-oxygenase (also called PG synthetase), PG and other products are formed. PG have molecular weights between 300 and 400 and contain only carbon, hydrogen, and oxygen atoms. They are identified by the letters A to I. The number of substitutions on the ring is important, shown by the letters A or B (oxygen), D or E (oxygen and hydroxyl), and F (two hydroxyl groups). PGG and PGH are unstable intermediate endoperoxides ($T_{\frac{1}{2}} = 5$ min in aqueous media) that are converted to stable PG, and PGI_2 is named prostacyclin. Greek letters α or β (e.g., PGF_{β}) show the spatial orientation of the hydroxyl group at carbon 9 on the cyclo-pentane ring. Most naturally occurring PG are of the α type. The biological properties of each PG differ according to the number of double bonds in the chain, which are indicated by subscript numerals 1, 2, and 3. The structures of some of the products of the arachidonic acid cascade, including prostanoic acid, the structure common to all PG, are shown in Figure 2. Under certain conditions, the action of both the endoperoxides and PG in inflammation may be important, since they affect smooth muscles, blood vessels, and nerve cells.

A compound with a short half-life ($T_{\frac{1}{2}} = 30$ sec) was isolated from products of arachidonic acid metabolism in human platelets (thrombocytes) (33,34). This acid lipid with oxane structure caused platelet aggregation and the constriction of arteries; since it was first found in thrombocytes, it was called a thromboxane(s). It also is a product of the conversion of endoperoxides by cyclo-oxygenase. Each compound is named by a capital letter (e.g., thromboxane A_2) that signifies the basic structure of the compound. The subscript arabic numeral indicates the number of double bonds, as in the nomenclature for PG. After the isolation of thromboxane(s) in platelets, they were found in many different tissues and cells. Under certain physiological conditions, they may play a more important role in inflammation than do PG. Thromboxane A_2 is converted to the stable but inactive thromboxane B_2.

Another product in the arachidonic acid pathway has been isolated and called prostacyclin (PGI_2) (35). This substance is also derived from endoperoxides. It is produced principally by endothelial cells, has vasodilatory action, inhibits platelet aggregation, and increases the concentration of cyclic adenosine monophosphate (cAMP) in certain cells. The concept that has emerged with these compounds is that thromboxanes and prostacyclins mediate vascular tone and thrombogenesis because of their antagonistic activities.

Other products of arachidonic acid oxidation, but via the

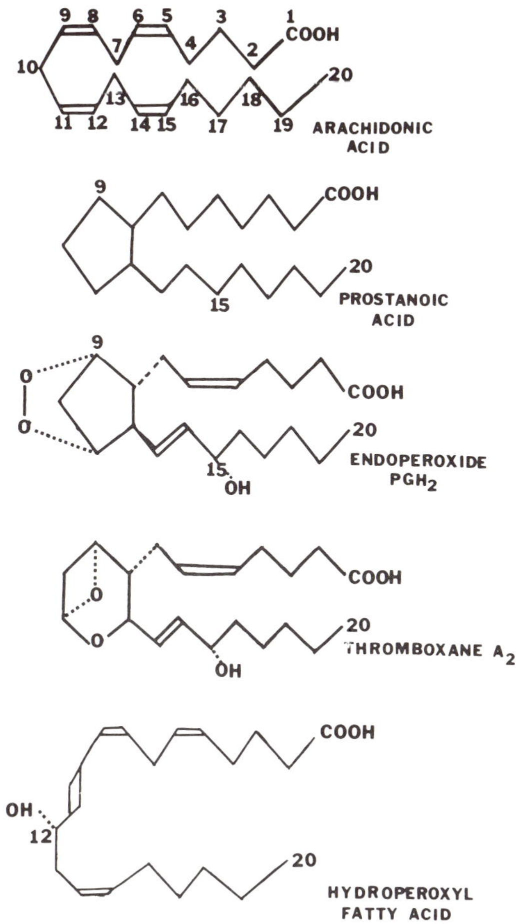

FIGURE 2

Structure of arachidonic acid and some of its oxidation products. Prostanoic acid is the basic structure of all prostaglandins.

lipooxygenase pathway, include leukotrienes and hydroperoxyl fatty acids. Leukotrienes are produced mainly by leukocytes and also are known as the slow reactive substance of anaphylaxis, SRS-A (36). The lipooxygenase pathway is differentiated from the reactions involving cyclo-oxygenase because this pathway is not inhibited by aspirin (see following).

Therefore, the current concept is that cellular phospholipids are released by promoters of inflammation. Arachidonic acid, a polyunsaturated fatty acid (Fig. 2), is released by the action of a widespread phospholipase that acts on the phospholipids. The arachidonic acid is oxidized enzymatically (cyclo-oxygenase or lipooxygenase) or nonenzymatically (UV irradiation or free radical products derived from oxygen) to endoperoxides, thromboxanes, prostacyclin, the various PG, leukotrienes, and hydroperoxyl fatty acids. Many of these products have a role in the inflammatory process. Since they are all short-lived, they are most effective near sites of production.

PG of the E group have been investigated as mediators of inflammation for a number of years. They promote erythema and exacerbate edema and pain caused by other mediators such as bradykinin and histamine. The first studies of infusion of PGE_1 in human beings were done in 1959; this resulted in an increase in heart rate and a slight fall in arterial blood pressure (37). Activity similar to that of PG was found in inflammatory exudates (38); during phagocytosis PG are released from PMN-leukocytes. PG may cause wheal and flare reactions and are released in trauma and shock. PGE_1 and PGE_2 cause local vascular leakage when injected into human and animal skin (39–41). Both cause edema formation similar to, or together with, bradykinin and histamine (42,43). In addition, arachidonic acid is chemotactic for PMN-leukocytes. This activity is greatly enhanced when the fatty acid is exposed to UV light, hydrogen peroxide, or superoxide anion (44,45). Thromboxane A_2 also has chemotactic properties, as do some of the products of lipooxygenase on arachidonic acid, including the fatty acids hydroperoxyeicosatetraenoic acid and hydroxyeicosatetraenoic acid (46,47). The structure of the latter compound is shown in Figure 2. The chemotactic properties of these compounds may account, in part, for some of the leukocyte migration to sites of inflammation and tissue injury in various connective tissue diseases. The action of these substances in producing some of the cardinal features of inflammation is discussed in more detail in Weissmann (31).

In in vitro experiments, the entire wide variety of nonsteroidal anti-inflammatory drugs appears to inhibit PG synthesis (48). At the level of the microsome, the enzyme cyclo-oxygenase catalyzes the conversion of some of the essential polyunsaturated fatty acids into the endoperoxides, which in turn are converted to PG, thromboxanes, and other products (Fig. 2). It is the cyclo-oxygenase that is inhibited by all noncorticosteroidal antiinflammatory drugs such as aspirin, indomethacin, phenylbutazone, mefenamic acid, meclofenamic acid, flufenamic acid, and naproxen. An additional action of aspirin is the acetylation of the active site of cyclo-oxygenase. The other agents just mentioned probably have additional activities as well.

Antiinflammatory glucocorticoids such as cortisol, prednisolone, and betamethasone do not inhibit PG synthetase. However, at least one of their activities is to inhibit a step prior to the formation of arachidonic acid, such as blocking the access of membrane phospholipid to phospholipase (49) or directly inhibiting the action of the phospholipase (50). When this occurs, little or no polyunsaturated fatty acids are available as substrates for cyclo-oxygenase.

There are a number of other drugs commonly used for diseases characterized by acute and chronic inflammation. Their affects on PG synthesis have been investigated. Gold salts inhibited PG synthesis. This was shown in patients with pemphigus receiving systemic chrysotherapy (51). D-penicillamine had no affect on cyclo-oxygenase, but may cause inhibition of certain PG because of its action as a metal-chelating agent. Copper is required as a cofactor for the synthesis of PG (52). Experiments with the antimalarial drugs on the synthesis of PG have given variable results, although interference has been noted in some reports (32). Finally, studies of the interrelationship(s) of these arachidonic acid oxidation pathway products with other mediator systems implicated in the inflammatory process are still in their infancy. This will be a fertile field of study for the future.

LYSOSOMAL ENZYMES

The cellular response in an acute inflammatory exudate is mediated by biochemical and immunologic reactions that cause the mobilization, leukotaxis, and localization of PMN-leukocytes at sites of injury (53). Other cell types involved in the reaction include tissue mast cells, wandering and fixed macrophages, platelets, lymphocytes, and fibroblasts involved in tissue repair. The events that cause the cellular response are due, in part, to the action of a number of different factors: C5a, $C\overline{5,6,7}$, and Ba in the complement system, possibly arachidonic acid and/or its oxidation products (see the earlier discussion of prostaglandins), and Factor XII, which in turn activate the kinin, fibrinolytic, and blood clotting systems. All these pathways produce specific cleavage products that may elicit a chemotactic response.

Central to this theme is the degranulation of lysosomes of accumulated PMN leukocytes and the release of enzymes and other factors that play an important role in both the evolution and subsequent tissue injury characteristic of the inflammatory response (54,55). Substrates for these enzymes include connective tissue proteoglycan, collagen, vascular basement membranes, and the elastic walls of arteries and venules (54–56). More than 25 enzymes and other factors have been identified in lysosomes. These include organophosphorus-resistant esterases, arylsulfatase, β-glucuronidase, neutral and acid cathepsins, collagenase (57), and elastase (58). In reference to the tissue destruction in inflammation, there are four important proteases: elastase, collagenase, cathepsin D, and cathepsin G (59,60). The hydrolysis of collagen by collagenase and proteoglycan by cathepsin D are followed by the action of cathepsin G and elastase on both substrates.

These events result in further leukocyte accumulation and release of lysosomal constituents and even greater tissue damage (61). Thus PMN leukocyte chemotaxis and accumulation is self-perpetuating. In rheumatoid arthritis, the accumulation and lysis of the leukocytes in joint spaces are probably responsible for much of the cutaneous and joint inflammation and cartilage degradation. Other cells that contribute to the inflammatory changes of arthritis by releasing lysosomal enzymes include synovial lining cells, chondrocytes, and mononuclear cells. Eventually, because of the continuous damage to joint cells and tissues, the arthritis may become chronic with focal collections of lymphocytes, pannus formation with cartilage destruction, joint erosion, and synovial hyperplasia and necrosis. Mononuclear cells predominate at this time. Both gamma globulin and complement components are synthesized in situ in joints (62,63), and kinins have been identified in rheumatoid joint fluid. Thus these sites are probably a constant source of immune globulins as well as complement-, kinin-, arachidonic acid-, and fibrin-derived chemotactic factors.

If antigen-antibody complexes provoked the inflammation, as in some types of glomerulonephritis, the accumulated PMN leukocytes may undergo phagocytosis. The complexes, via the Fc portion of the immunoglobulin and C3b and/or C3d (cleavage products of native C3; see the first chapter on the Complement System), bind to the phagocytic cells, causing the release of the contents of the lysosomes. In addition, PMN-leukocytes undergoing phagocytosis release the oxidation products of arachidonic acid (prostaglandins, thromboxanes), which are potent mediators of inflammation. The formation of these products is enhanced by the production of derivatives of molecular oxygen during phagocytosis: O_2^- (superoxide anion); H_2O_2, and OH^- (hydroxyl radicals).

At least one of the mechanisms of antiinflammatory steroids such as cortisone, prednisolone, and cortisol is to stabilize lysosomes and to increase their resistance to rupture (64). The nonsteroidal antiinflammatory drugs such as aspirin and indomethacin do not affect the release of lysosomal granules.

REFERENCES

1. Movat H, Broklehurst WE. Pharmacological mediators of immediate hypersensitivity: II. Plasma factors. In: Brent L, Holborow J, eds. Progress in Immunology II, Vol. 4. Amsterdam: North-Holland, p. 298, 1974.
2. Ryan GB. Inflammation: mediators of inflammation. Beitr Pathol 152:272-291, 1974.
3. Cochrane CG, Revak SD, Ulevitch R, Johnston AJ, Morrison D. Hageman factor: characterization and mechanism of activation. In: Pisano JJ, Austen KF, eds. Chemistry and Biology of the Kallikrein-Kinin System in Health and Disease. Washington, DC: US Government Printing Office, p. 17, 1976.
4. Mandle R Jr, Kaplan AP. Hageman factor substrates: Human prekallikrein: Mechanism of activation by Hageman factor and participation in Hageman factor-dependent fibrinolysis. J Biol Chem 252:6097-6104, 1977.
5. Alving BM, Hojima Y, Pisano JJ, et al. Hypotension associated with prekallikrein activator (Hageman-factor fragments) in plasma protein fraction. N Engl J Med 299:66-77, 1978.
6. Griffin JH, Cochrane CG. Recent advances in the understanding of contact activation reactions. Semin Thromb Hemostas 5:254, 1979.
7. Gigli I, Mason JW, Colman RW, et al. Interaction of plasma kallikrein with the C1 inhibitor. J Immunol 104:574-581, 1970.
8. Cochrane CG, Revak SD, Wuepper, KD. Activation of Hageman factor in solid and fluid phases. J Exp Med 138:1564-1583, 1973.
9. Kaplan AP, Austen KF. A prealbumin activator of prekallikrein: II. Derivation of activators of prekallikrein from active Hageman factor by digestion with plasmin. J Exp Med 133:696-712, 1971.
10. Nagasawa S, Takahashi H, Koida M, et al. Partial purification of bovine plasma kallikreinogen, its activation by the Hageman factor. Biochem Biophys Res Commun 32:644-699, 1968.

11. Damus PS, Hicks M, Rosenberg RD. Anticoagulant action of heparin. Nature 246:355-357, 1973.
12. Heck LW, Kaplan AP. Substrates of Hageman factor: I. Isolation and characterization of human factor XI (PTA) and inhibition of the activated enzyme by α1-antitrypsin. J Exp Med 140:1615-1630, 1974.
13. Schachter M. Kallikreins and kinins. Physiol Rev 49:509-547, 1969.
14. Wilhelm DL. Kinins in human disease. Ann Rev Med 22:63-84, 1971.
15. Kaplan, AP, Kay AB, Austen KF. A prealbumin activator of prekallikrein: III. Appearance of chemotactic activity for human neutrophils by the conversion of human prekallikrein to kallikrein. J Exp Med 135:81-97, 1972.
16. Saito H, Man-Chiu P, Vicic W, Goldsmith GH Jr, Menitove JE. Human plasma prekallikrein (Fletcher factor) clotting activity and antigen in health and disease. J Lab Clin Med 92:84-95, 1978.
17. Blomback B, Blomback M, Edman P, et al. Human fibrinopeptides, isolation, characterization, and structure. Biochem Biophys Acta 115:371-396, 1966.
18. Kay AB, Pepper DS, Ewert MR. Generation of chemotactic activity for leukocytes by the action of thrombin on human fibrinogen. Nature (New Biol) 243:56-57.
19. Starzl TE, Dixon FJ. Clotting changes, including disseminated intravascular coagulation, during rapid renal-homograft rejection. N Engl J Med 282:383, 1970.
20. Nussenzweig V, Seligmann M, Pelmont J, et al. Les produits de degradation du fibrinogene humain par la plasmine: I. Separation et proprietes physiochimiques. Ann Inst Pasteur Lille 100:377-389, 1971.
21. Lewis JH, Wilson JH. Fibrinogen breakdown products. Am J Physiol 207:1053-1057, 1964.
22. Fletcher AP, Alkjaersig N, Fisher S, et al. The proteolysis of fibrinogen by plasmin: the identification of thrombin-clottable fibrinogen derivatives which polymerize abnormally. J Lab Clin Med 68:780-802, 1966.
23. Nilehn JE. Split products of fibrinogen after prolonged interaction with plasmin. Thromb Diath Haemorrh 18:89-100, 1967.
24. Triantaphyllopoulos E, Triantaphyllopoulos DC. Micromolecular fragments split from fibrinogen. Thromb Diath Haemorrh 18:300-301, 1967.
25. Sherry S. Fibrinolytic agents. In: Dowling HF, ed. Disease-a-Month. Chicago: Year Book Medical Publishers, May 1969, p. 1.
26. Marder VJ, Shulman NR, Carrol WR. High molecular weight derivatives of human fibrinogen produced by plasmin: I. Physicochemical and immunological characterization. J Biol Chem 244:2111-2119, 1969.
27. Bergstrom S. Isolation, structure, and action of the prostaglandins. In: Bergstrom S, Samuelsson B, eds. Prostaglandins. Proceedings, II Nobel Symposium. Stockholm: Almqvist and Wiksell, 1967, p. 21.
28. Bergstrom S. Prostaglandins: members of a new hormonal system. Science 157:382-391, 1967.

29. Samuelsson B. Biosynthesis and metabolism of prostaglandins. Prog Biochem Pharmacol 3:59, 1967.
30. Lands W, Lee R, Smith W. Factors regulating the biosynthesis of various prostaglandins. Ann NY Acad Sci 180:107, 1971.
31. Weissmann G. Prostaglandins in acute inflammation. Current Concepts (Upjohn Company), 1980.
32. Trang LE. Prostaglandins and inflammation. Semin Arthritis Rheum 9:153-190, 1980.
33. Hamberg M, Svensson J, Samuelsson B. Thromboxanes: a new group of biologically active compounds derived from prostaglandin endoperoxides. Proc Natl Acad Sci 72:2994-2998, 1975.
34. Samuelsson B, Paoletti R. Advances in Prostaglandin and Thromboxane Research. New York: Raven Press, Vol. 1, 1976.
35. Moncada S, Gryglewski R, Bunting S. Vane JR. A enzyme isolated from arteries transforms prostaglandin endoperoxides to an unstable substance that inhibits platelet aggregation. Nature 263:663-665, 1976.
36. Borgeat P, Samuelsson B. Arachidonic acid metabolism in polymorphonuclear leukocytes: effects of ionophore A23187. Proc Natl Acad Sci 76:2148-2152, 1979.
37. Bergstrom S, Duner H, von Euler US, et al. Observations on the effects of infusion of prostaglandin E in man. Acta Physiol Scand 45:145-151, 1959.
38. Willis AL. In: Mantegazza P, Horton EW, eds. Prostaglandins, Peptides, and Amines. New York: Academic Press, 1969, p. 31.
39. Higgs GA, Youlten LJF. Prostaglandin production by rabbit peritoneal polymorphonuclear leukocytes in vitro. Br J Pharmacol 44:330, 1972.
40. Crunkhorn P, Willis AL. Cutaneous reactions to intradermal prostaglandins. Br J Pharmacol 41:49-56, 1971.
41. Kaley G, Weiner R. Prostaglandin E_1: a potential mediator of the inflammatory response. Ann NY Acad Sci 180:338-350, 1971.
42. Moncada S, Ferreira SH, Vane JR. Prostaglandins, aspirin-like drugs, and oedema of inflammation. Nature 246:217-219, 1973.
43. Williams TJ, Morley J. Prostaglandins as potentiators of increased vascular permeability in inflammation. Nature 246:215-217, 1973.
44. Turner SR, Campbell JA, Lynn WS. Polymorphonuclear chemotaxis toward oxidized lipid components of cell membranes. J Exp Med 141:1437-1441, 1975.
45. Perez HD, Weksler B, Goldstein I. A new mechanism for the generation of biologically active products from arachidonic acid. Clin Res 27:464A, 1979.
46. Kitchen EA, Boot JR, Dawson W. Chemotactic activity of thromboxane A_2 for polymorphonuclear leukocytes. Prostaglandins 16:239-244, 1978.
47. Goetzl EJ, Gorman RR. Chemotactic and chemokinetic stimulation of human eosinophil and neutrophil polymorphonuclear leukocytes by 12-L-hydroxy-5,8,10-heptadecatrienoic acid (HHT). J Immunol 120:526-531, 1978.

48. Vane JR. The mode of action of aspirin-like drugs. Agents Actions 8:430–431, 1978.
49. Hong SL, Levine L. Inhibition of arachidonic acid release from cells as the biochemical action of antiinflammatory corticosteroids. Proc Natl Acad Sci 73:1730–1734, 1976.
50. Flower RJ. Steroidal antiinflammatory drugs as inhibitors of phospholipase A_2. In: Galli C, Galli G, Porcellati G, eds. Advances in Prostaglandin and Thromboxane Research. New York: Raven Press, 1978, Vol 3, p. 105.
51. Pennys NS, Ziboh V, Gottlieb NL, et al. Inhibition of prostaglandin synthesis and human epidermal enzymes by aurothiomalate in vitro: possible actions of gold in pemphigus. J Invest Dermatol 63:356–361, 1974.
52. Maddox IS. The role of copper in prostaglandin synthesis. Biochim Biophys Acta 306:74–81, 1973.
53. Hersh EM, Bodey GP. Leukocytic mechanisms in inflammation. Annu Rev Med 21:105–132, 1970.
54. Cochrane CG. Immunologic tissue injury mediated by neutrophilic leukocytes. Adv Immunol 9:97–162, 1968.
55. McKay DG. Participation of components of the blood coagulation system in the inflammatory response. Am J Pathol 67:181–203, 1972.
56. Weissmann G. The many-faceted lysosome. In: Good RA, Fisher DW, eds. Immunobiology. Stanford, CA: Sinauer Assoc, 1971, p. 37.
57. Lazarus GS, Daniels JR, Brown RS, et al. Degradation of collagen by a human granulocyte collagenolytic system. J Clin Invest 47:2622–2629, 1968.
58. Janoff A, Scherer J. Mediators of inflammation in leukocyte lysosomes: IX. Elastinolytic activity in granules of human polymorphonuclear leukocytes. J Exp Med 128:1137–1155, 1968.
59. Weissmann G, Smolen JE, Hoffstein S. Polymorphonuclear leukocytes as secretory organs of inflammation. J Invest Dermatol 71:95–99, 1978.
60. Weissmann G, Korchak HM, Perez HD, Smolen JE, Goldstein IM, Hoffstein ST. Leukocytes as secretory organs of inflammation. In: Weissmann G, Paoletti R, Samuelsson B, eds. Advances in Inflammation Research. New York: Raven Press, 1979.
61. Borel, JF, Keller HU, Sorkin E. Studies on chemotaxis: XI. Effect on neutrophils of lysosomal and other subcellular fractions from leukocytes. Int Arch Allergy Appl Immunol 35:194–205, 1969.
62. Smiley JD, Sachs C, Ziff M. In vitro synthesis of immunoglobulin by rheumatoid synovial membrane. J Clin Invest 47:624–632, 1968.
63. Ruddy S, Colten HR. Rheumatoid arthritis: biosynthesis of complement proteins by synovial tissues. N Engl J. Med 290:1284–1288, 1974.
64. Dunham P, Babiarz P, Israel A, Zerial A, Weissmann G. Membrane fusion: studies with a calcium-sensitive dye, Arsen azo III, in liposomes. Proc Natl Acad Sci 74:1580–1584, 1977.

SYNOVIANALYSIS

NORMAN L. GOTTLIEB, M.D.

Synovianalysis, serologic studies, and roentgenograms form the critical cluster of tests used in evaluating rheumatic disorders (1). Because synovial fluid composition reflects articular pathology, synovianalysis is important diagnostically and expands our knowledge and understanding of relevant pathophysiologic events. Analysis of joint fluid is a vital part of the workup of every patient with undefined arthritis. Frequently it is helpful in monitoring disease course or response to treatment. Clinicians treating rheumatic conditions should be familiar with the tests that are available and should develop skills in their interpretation.

TECHNIQUE OF JOINT ASPIRATION

Knowledge of joint anatomy and neighboring structures is essential for the proper aspiration technique. The various approaches to individual joints illustrated in standard texts will not be reviewed. Aseptic technique is mandatory; disposable needles and syringes reduce the danger of infection. Following cleansing of the injection site with a topical antiseptic, the skin is sprayed with ethyl chloride. A 10-cc syringe with a 20-gauge needle is adequate for removal of all but the most tenacious fluids. Lidocaine may be infiltrated into the skin and deeper tissues for local anesthesia. All recoverable fluid should be removed with each aspiration. Following arthrocentesis the skin is dried with a cotton pledget and a bandage is applied. Patients are permitted to return to their former level of activity upon completion of the procedure unless joint rest is indicated by the disease process.

The knees are tapped most frequently, but most other large joints

TABLE 1
The Results of Synovianalysis in Different Forms of Arthritis

Group	Disease	Color	Clarity	Viscosity	Mucin clot
Group I noninflammatory	Normal	Straw	Transparent	High	Good
	Traumatic arthritis	Straw to bloody to xantho-chromic	Transparent to turbid	High	Good
	Osteoarthritis	Yellow	Transparent	High	Good
	Systemic lupus erythemato-sus (SLE)	Straw	Slightly cloudy	High	Good
Group II inflammatory	Rheumatic fever	Yellow	Slightly cloudy	Low	Good
	Pseudogout	Yellow	Slightly cloudly (if acute)	Low (if acute)	Good to poor
	Gout	Yellow to milky	Cloudy	Low	Poor
	Rheumatoid arthritis	Yellow to greenish	Cloudy	Low	Poor
Group III septic	Tuberculous arthritis	Yellow	Cloudy	Low	Poor
	Septic arthritis	Grayish or bloody	Turbid purulent	Low	Poor

*"RA" cells: Rheumatoid cells are not morphologically specific, but these inclusion-bearing cells are most frequently seen in high concentration in rheumatoid arthritis.

†"LE" cells may be demonstrated in Wright-stained smears of sediment from centrifuged synovial fluid in SLE.

From Hollander JL, McCarty DJ Jr, eds. Arthritis and Allied Conditions, 1972. Courtesy of Lea & Febiger.

and many small ones are accessible to the skilled practitioner. The hip joint, being deep and adjacent to vital structures, is technically more difficult to aspirate.

The combined experience from many clinics has shown the incidence of Iatrogenic joint infection following aspiration to be less than 1 case in 7000 procedures. Joints should not be aspirated if there is infection of the skin or subcutaneous tissues or in the presence of uncontrolled bleeding diathesis.

Table 1 (*continued*)

Cell WBC/mm³; % Polys	Cartilage debris	Crystals	"RA" cells*	Bacteria
<200 WBC; <25	0	0	0	0
<2000 WBC; few to many RBC; <25	0 or +	0	0	0
1000 WBC; <25	+	0	0	0
5000 WBC; 10	0	0	0†	0
10,000 WBC to 12,000; 50	0	0	0 or +	0
1000 to 5000 WBC; 25 to 50	+	Calcium pyrophosphate	0	0
10,000 to 12,000 WBC; 60 to 70	0	Urate +	0	0
15,000 to 20,000 WBC; 75	0	Occasional cholesterol	+	0
25,000 WBC; 50 to 60	0	0	0	+
80 to 200,000; 75	0	0	0	+

NORMAL SYNOVIAL FLUID

The constituents of synovial fluid are derived by dialysis from the plasma and by synthesis from synovial cells, which manufacture the mucopolysaccharide, hyaluronate (2). Small molecules tend to be in similar concentrations in blood and joint fluid (e.g., uric acid), whereas large polymers (e.g., blood proteins) are in lesser quantity in synovial fluid. Fibrinogen, prothrombin, Factors V and VII, and other hemostatis constituents are not normally present, which accounts for failure of synovial fluid to clot (Table 1).

Normal synovial fluid is slightly alkaline, clear yellow, and viscous like egg white. The cell count is usually less than 200/mm³ and predominantly mononuclear leukocytes. The quantity of fluid present depends upon joint size and the patient's age. Glucose content is similar to that in blood if fasting specimens are obtained. There is approximately 33% as much protein in synovial fluid as in whole blood, of which 60% is albumin. Hyaluronate concentration is 0.3 g/dl.

SYNOVIAL FLUID EXAMINATION

Following arthrocentesis, the gross appearance, quantity, color, and clarity of the fluid should be recorded. An accurate estimate of viscosity may be obtained by a string test, which is performed by allowing the fluid to drip slowly from a syringe or by placing a drop of fluid on the index finger and thumb and then separating the digits. Normally, the string will be greater than 4 cm before breaking. Viscosity, essentially a function of hyaluronate, increases exponentially relative to increasing concentrations of hyaluronate. Reduced viscosity may be obtained by precipitating the hyaluronate with various acids, by hydrolytic degradation with certain enzymes, or by physical processes, such as ultrasound. Synovial fluid viscosity usually is lower with inflammatory arthropathies.

The mucin clot, or Ropes' test, similarly is dependent on hyaluronate content and character. Several drops of 5% acetic acid are added to a few ml of synovial fluid in a test tube, causing the protein-polysaccharide complex (mucin) to precipitate. In normal and osteoarthritic fluids a firm clot forms that will not separate or shed on shaking. In rheumatoid arthritis (RA), gout, and septic arthritis, hyaluronate polymerization usually is decreased and only a cloudy solution forms or a friable clot appears that will fracture upon shaking. Fluids that exhibit poor viscosity generally form poor mucin clots.

The number of leukocytes per mm^3 may be determined in a counting chamber, with isotonic saline substituted for the usual counting fluid. Most arthritic conditions are associated with a leukocytosis; the more acute the state, the greater the number of polymorphonuclear leukocytes present.

Synovial fluid glucose determination should be performed while fasting, as there is a normal delay in glucose equilibrium between the vascular and articular compartments. A simultaneous blood glucose determination should be obtained. Markedly decreased synovial fluid glucose values are commonly found in septic processes; but some inflammatory arthritides also may have decreased levels.

Gram stains and bacterial and fungal cultures should be obtained whenever infectious arthritis is suspected clinically. Microbial antigens may sometimes be detected by countercurrent immunoelectrophoresis, a recently developed technique that is particularly useful with pneumococcal infection.

Rheumatoid factor may be measured in synovial fluid or in the extract of synovial cells using the same technique as for serum. Little additional information is derived from this test, however, as rheumatoid factor usually is absent in the joint when absent also in the blood.

Microscopic examination should be performed using a drop of fresh, uncentrifuged fluid placed on a clean slide and enclosed with a cover slip. Crystals of various types (3,4), sodium urate, calcium pyrophosphate, cholesterol, oxalate, and hydroxyapatitic and steroids may be identified (Figs. 1 and 2). Cartilage fragments, collagen fibrils, cytoplasmic inclusion granules, fibrin strands, macrophages, and synovial cells frequently are observed.

FIGURE 1

Multiple intracellular rhomboid-shaped calcium pyrophosphate crystals in synovial fluid aspirated from the knee of an elderly male with chondrocalcinosis and pseudogout.

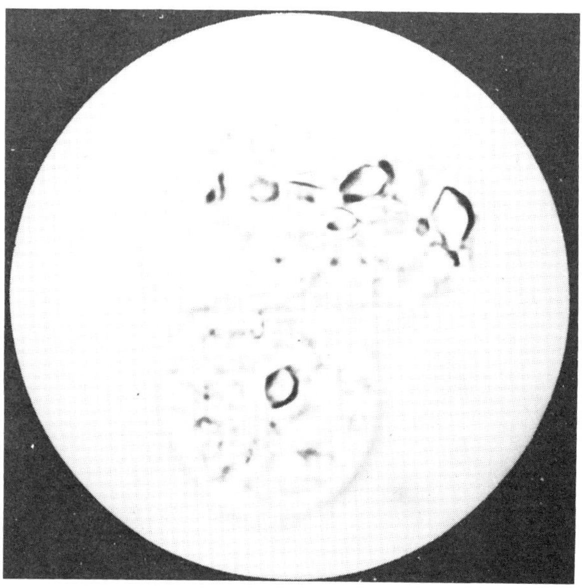

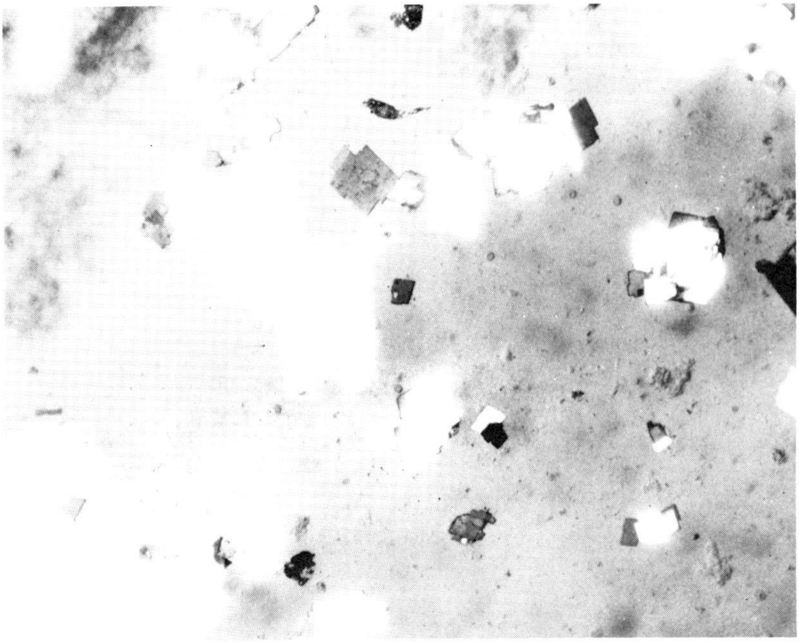

FIGURE 2
Cholesterol crystals are found in the synovial fluid of a small percentage of patients with rheumatoid arthritis and other rheumatic disorders.

Joint fluid hemolytic complement levels may be elevated in Reiter's syndrome and depressed in RA, systemic lupus erythematosus (SLE), septic arthritis, and, rarely, crystal deposition disease.

SYNOVIAL FLUID FINDINGS IN DISEASE STATES

Gout

Gouty synovial fluid most commonly is greenish-yellow and turbid, although it may be clear, chalky, bloody, or even purulent. The white blood cell count ranges from 1000 to 70,000/mm^3 or more, with a mean of about 15,000 cells mm^3. During the acute attack, polymorphonuclear leukocytes predominate. Both the mucin clot and the string sign usually are poor. Glucose levels most often are in the normal range.

The identification of sodium urate crystals, which usually appear as needle-shaped rods, by microscopic examination of fresh unstained synovial fluid is possible in most cases (5). Often they are seen within a few moments, but at times a 15-min search is necessary. Crystals may be intra- and/or extracellular; during acute gouty attacks a greater proportion are intracellular. Monosodium urate monohydrate (MSU) crystals are identified with certainty by compensated polarized light microscopy; they appear strongly birefringent and optically negative.

A number of other substances may be confused with sodium urate crystals because of similar appearance. Calcium pyrophosphate crystals, fibrin, collagen fibrils, and various steroid crystals from previous intraarticular injections are the commonest cause of false positive identification.

Calcium Pyrophosphate Arthropathy (Pseudogout)

Pseudogout is another crystal-induced arthritis that may be diagnosed by microscopic examination of unstained synovial fluid. Calcium pyrophosphate dihydrate (CPPD) crystals have several distinct forms (6). Most common is the rhomboid shape, but needles, rods, or fragments of many configurations may be found intra- or extracellularly. The finding of rhomboid crystals is most helpful as this differentiates pseudogout from gout morphologically.

Calcium phosphate crystals may be distinguished from MSU or orthophosphate (dicalcium phosphate dihydrate) and apatite crystals by several methods including polarizing light microscopy (CPPD crystals are positively birefringent), x-ray diffraction, and scanning electron microscopy and electron probe microanalysis. Chemical methods for differentiating MSU and CPPD crystals include the addition of uricase, which digests only urate crystals, and increasing the pH to 9, which dissolves urate but not pyrophosphate crystals.

Reiter's Syndrome

Two features of synovial fluid examination are sometimes helpful in diagnosing Reiter's syndrome. The first is an elevated hemolytic complement (C′) level, which usually is greater than 140 $C'H_{50}$ units. In one study, the mean complement level in Reiter's syndrome was 170 units, compared with 43 units in RA and 102 units in gout. Reasons for synovial complement elevation are unclear, but they may relate to higher blood complement levels (325 units in Reiter's syndrome, 200 in RA, 280 in gout). The second finding is that of giant macrophages containing numerous vacuoles and cytoplasmic granules and one or more intact polymorphonuclear leukocytes. These cells are infrequent (1 to 3% of the total leukocyte population) and are not pathognomonic, being found in several joint diseases.

Rheumatoid Arthritis

Although the synovial fluid findings in RA are nondiagnostic, several features support the diagnosis. RA cells, or ragocytes, are polymorphonuclear leukocytes with cytoplasmic inclusions that occur in 5 to 95% of the total white cell population. These inclusions consist of gamma globulin-rheumatoid factor complexes, as shown by cell maceration or fluorescent-staining techniques. Cells of identical morphologic appearance have been found in numerous other arthritides, however.

A poor mucin clot is a characteristic of RA, although many rheumatoid fluids will clot normally. The importance of a poor mucin clot diagnostically is shown by its inclusion in the American Rheumatism Association's criteria for the diagnosis of RA (see Table 1 of the next chapter on Rheumatoid Arthritis).

Infrequently, cholesterol crystals are seen in rheumatoid synovial fluid. They are readily identified by their distinctive morphology, being rhomboid-shaped with one or more corner notches. Their significance is unclear, but often they are found in severe disease of long duration.

Rheumatoid factor can be demonstrated in synovial fluid and synovial cell extract. Whereas most patients have rheumatoid factor in serum and synovial fluid in varying titers, the synovial fluid will be positive and the serum negative in a few patients. This may be a clue to the early diagnosis of RA.

Synovial fluid $C'H_{50}$ commonly is depressed in seropositive RA, whereas the serum complement level usually is normal or slightly increased.

Traumatic Arthritis

Synovial fluid from a traumatized joint may be clear, turbid, serosanguineous, or grossly bloody. Usually, less than 2000 white blood cells per mm^3 are present. The number of red blood cells varies widely;

viscosity and mucin clot are normal. A bloodly fluid is not diagnostic of traumatic arthritis and may be encountered with bleeding diatheses (especially hemophilia), tumors, pigmented villonodular synovitis, and neuropathic joint disease. Streaks of bright red blood in the apsirate usually are indicative of traumatic tap.

Septic Arthritis

A definitive diagnosis of septic arthritis is established by the identification of microorganisms in synovial fluid on gram stain by growth in culture. In some instances of almost certain infection, these tests are negative. False positive results may be caused by contamination.

Additional findings supporting this diagnosis include puslike appearance, white blood cell count greater than 50,000/mm^3, and depressed glucose level. However, these findings may be absent in gonococcal arthritis and are less commonly found with other nonvirulent organisms. On occasion, synovial fluid leukocytosis in noninfectious inflammatory joint disease (e.g., RA, crystal-induced arthritis), may be extreme, causing diagnostic confusion (7).

Degenerative Joint Disease

Fluid from an osteoarthritic joint generally is light yellow or honey-colored and transparent. Few white blood cells are present, viscosity is good, string sign is 4 cm or longer, and a firm clot is formed upon addition of acetic acid. Often, cartilage fragments and collagen fibrils will be seen on microscopic examination.

In severe degenerative disease, or when inflammation is superimposed, an entirely different galaxy of findings may emerge. The synovial fluid may then resemble that of rheumatoid or traumatic arthritis.

REFERENCES

1. McCarty DJ. Synovial fluid. In: McCarty DJ, ed. Arthritis and Allied Conditions. Philadelphia: Lea & Febiger 1979, 9th ed, p. 51.
2. Ropes MW, Bauer W. Synovial Fluid Changes in Joint Disease. Cambridge, MA: Harvard University Press, 1953.
3. Hollander JL. Arthrocentesis and intrasynovial therapy. In: Hollander JL, McCarty DJ, eds. Arthritis and Allied Conditions. Philadelphia: Lea & Febiger, 9th ed., p. 402.

4. Zuckner J, Uddin J, Gantner GE, Dorner RW. Cholesterol crystals in synovial fluid. Ann Intern Med 60: 436–446, 1964.
5. McCarty DJ, Hollander JL. Identification of urate crystals in gouty synovial fluid. Ann Intern Med 54:452–460, 1961.
6. McCarty DJ, Kohn NN, Faires JS. Significance of calcium phosphate crystals in the synovial fluid of arthritic patients. The "pseudogout syndrome." Ann Intern Med 56:711–737, 1962.
7. Krey PR, Bailen DA. Synovial fluid leukocytosis: a study of extremes. Am J Med 67:436–442, 1979.

RHEUMATOID ARTHRITIS

NORMAN L. GOTTLIEB, M.D.

Rheumatoid arthritis (RA) is a systemic disease of unknown etiology involving primarily the diarthrodial joints but at times affecting most other organ systems. The course of this disorder is unpredictable and characterized by spontaneous remissions and exacerbations (1,2). Occasionally, the arthritis is mild and clears completely or remains confined to a few joints (pauciarticular).

The principal target organ of RA is the synovial membrane, which becomes infiltrated with inflammatory cells (predominantly lymphocytes and plasma cells), congested, and edematous; the synovial lining cells undergo hypertrophic and hyperplastic changes (3). With continued synovitis, a pannus of granulation tissue develops that sometimes extends over the surface of the cartilage and burrows into the subchondral bone causing cyst formation and erosions. In severe cases, large areas of bone are denuded of cartilage and adhesions form between joint surfaces, leading ultimately to fibrous or bony ankylosis. At other times, cartilage loss together with tendinous and ligamentous weakening results in instability or partial dislocation (subluxation).

EPIDEMIOLOGY

Surveys using the American Rheumatism Association criteria (Table 1) suggest that 2 to 6% of the adult U.S. population is affected. A female-to-male ratio of 2:1 or 3:1 is found, as is an increasing prevalence with age. The peak onset of RA is in the 20- to 40-year age group. Analysis of monozygotic twins, one of whom has RA, shows the disease is discordant. These findings, as well as those in American

TABLE 1
American Rheumatism Association Diagnostic Criteria*

1. Morning stiffness.
2. Pain on motion or tenderness in at least one joint (observed by a physician).
3. Swelling (soft tissue thickening or fluid, not bony overgrowth alone) in at least one joint (observed by a physician).
4. Swelling (observed by a physician) of at least one other joint (any interval free of joint symptoms between the two joint involvements may not be more than 3 months).
5. Symmetric joint swelling (observed by a physician) with simultaneous involvement of the same joint on both sides of the body (bilateral involvement of proximal interphalangeal, metacarpophalangeal, or metatarsophalangeal joints is acceptable without absolute symmetry). Terminal phalangeal joint involvement will not satisfy this criterion.
6. Subcutaneous nodules (observed by a physician) over bony prominences, on extensor surfaces, or in juxtaarticular regions.
7. Roentgenographic changes typical of rheumatoid arthritis (which must include at least bony decalcification localized to or most marked adjacent to the involved joints and not just degenerative changes). Degenerative changes do not exclude patients from any group classified as rheumatoid arthritis.
8. Positive agglutination test—demonstration of the "rheumatoid factor" by any method that, in two laboratories, has been positive in not more than 5% of normal controls.
9. Poor mucin precipitate from synovial fluid (with shreds and cloudy solution.
10. Characteristic histologic changes in synovium with three or more of the following: marked villous hypertrophy, proliferation of superficial synovial cells often with palisading, marked infiltration of chronic inflammatory cells (lymphocytes or plasma cells predominating) with tendency to form "lymphoid nodules," deposition of compact fibrin on the surface or interstitially, and foci of necrosis.
11. Characteristic histologic changes in subcutaneous nodules showing granulomatous foci with central zones of cell necrosis, surrounded by a palisade of proliferated macrophages and peripheral fibrosis, and chronic inflammatory cell infiltration, predominantly perivascular.

*The diagnosis of classic RA requires seven criteria: for items 1 through 5, joint symptoms or signs must be continuous for at least 6 weeks. The diagnosis of definite RA requires five of the above criteria, whereas probable RA requires three. In addition, there are 20 exclusions that must be met before the criteria are fulfilled.

Indian populations, have failed to provide evidence of genetic transmission. On the other hand, recent histocompatibility antigen studies show a sixfold increased prevalence of DR4 and DRW4 in RA patients, suggesting that a genetic factor may influence susceptibility to this illness. Attempts to define an infectious organism causally related to RA have failed.

CLINICAL FEATURES

In the adult, joint inflammation often is preceded by systemic manifestations such as fatigue, malaise, anorexia, weight loss, low grade fever, myalgias, and paresthesias. Disease onset usually is insidious with diffuse aching and stiffness not localized to joints. Frank articular pain, swelling, redness, warmth, tenderness, and limitation of function appear gradually. Morning stiffness is a frequent and prominent early complaint. Joint symptoms generally begin in the hands, especially the proximal interphalangeal (PIP) and metacarpophalangeal (MCP) joints, and feet, particularly the metatarsophalangeal (MTP) joints. Any diarthrodial joint may be involved singly or with multiple other joints, including the temporomandibular joints, the intervertebral facet joints, and the cricoarytenoid joints of the larnyx. Articular involvement tends to be symmetrical. Hemiparetic limbs frequently remain unaffected even with chronic active synovitis elsewhere. Tenosynovitis is frequent; extensor and flexor tendon sheaths about the wrists commonly are involved and may be associated with median nerve entrapment (carpal tunnel syndrome)

FIGURE 1
Prominent extensor tenosynovitis involving the dorsum of both wrists and hands in a female with active RA.

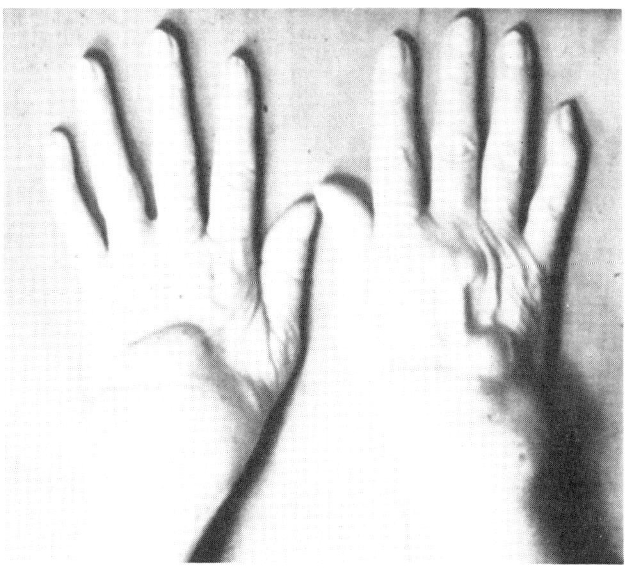

TABLE 2
Entrapment Neuropathies in RA

1. Median nerve
    a. Carpal tunnel syndrome
2. Ulnar nerve
    a. Cubital canal syndrome—elbow
    b. Canal of Guyon syndrome—wrist
3. Radial nerve
    a. Posterior interosseous syndrome
4. Sciatic nerve
    a. Tibial/common peroneal entrapment—Baker cyst
5. Posterior tibial nerve
    a. Tarsal tunnel syndrome
    b. Medial plantar syndrome
    c. Lateral plantar syndrome

(Fig. 1). Digital flexor tenosynovitis occurs in 50% of RA patients (4). Other entrapment neuropathies are listed in Table 2.

Joint deformities in part have their origin in muscle spasm, the flexors maintaining involuntary contraction with accompanying extensor relaxation. Inflammation and subsequent fibrosis of the capsule, ligaments, and musculotendinous apparatus lead to fixed deformities. Subluxation usually is preceded by cartilage and bone ero-

FIGURE 2
Dislocation of the second through fourth metacarpophalangeal joints, and a boutonniere deformity of the thumb, in RA of long duration.

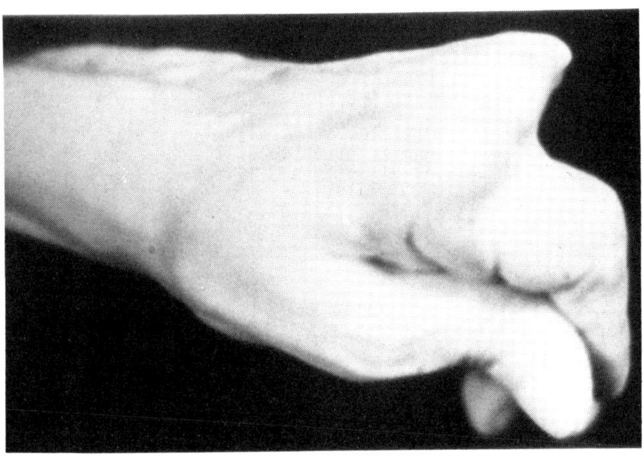

sion and destruction of supporting soft tissues, particularly ligaments and joint capsule. The most characteristic deformities in the RA hand are ulnar drift (ulnar deviation of the fingers), subluxation of the MCP joints, and fusiform swelling of the PIP joints. In the boutonniere deformity, the flexed PIP joint is forced through the extensor hood like a button through a hole, while the distal interphalangeal (DIP) joint is hyperextended (Fig. 2).

The swan-neck deformity is due to contraction of the intrinsic muscles of the hand producing hyperextension of the PIP joint and flexion of the DIP joint. Subluxation of the MTP joints and hallux valgus (bunion) formation lead to foot pain and difficulty in ambulating. Synovial cysts may complicate effusions of the knee (Baker's or popliteal cyst) and occasionally other joints. They generally connect with the joint space and originate as a herniation directly from the joint or

FIGURE 3

Extension-flexion views of the cervical spine showing C_1-C_2 subluxation, a common cause of neck pain in RA.

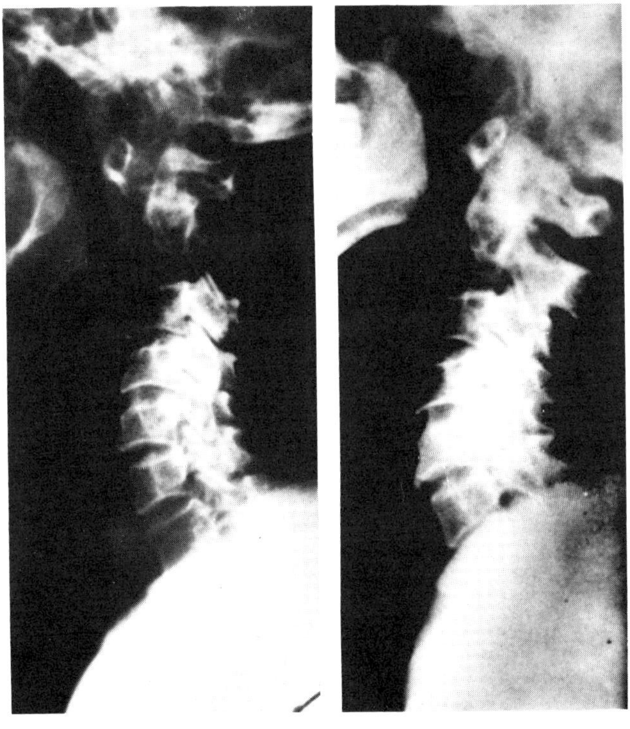

via a communicating bursa. Increased intraarticular pressure and distention of the joint capsule are thought to be responsible for cyst formation.

The atlantoaxial joints and other cervical vertebrae frequently are involved. Neck pain and limitation of motion and roentgenographic evidence of vertebral subluxation are common, but spinal cord compression with sensory and/or pyramidal tract signs are rare (Fig. 3).

EXTRAARTICULAR FEATURES

The extraarticular manifestations of RA are numerous and may be serious or life-threatening (5–7). Vasculitis is responsible for many, if not all, of the systemic features of RA (including the subcutaneous nodules). The terms "systemic" or "malignant" RA sometimes are used to denote the occurrence of rheumatoid vasculitis with target organ damage. The type and frequency of extraarticular features found in one group of 127 hospitalized Canadian patients, whose mean age and disease duration were 55 and 12 years, respectively, are shown in Table 3 (7). In this series, 34% of patients had one and 42% had two or more findings of extraarticular disease. The mortality rate was much higher in the presence of systemic illness, especially in patients above 50 years of age, infection contributing to the cause of death in 40% of cases.

Subcutaneous nodules eventually appear in approximately 25% of

TABLE 3
Extraarticular Findings

	%
Subcutaneous nodules	53
Pulmonary fibrosis	20
Digital vasculitis	15
Skin ulceration	13
Lymphadenopathy	12
Noncompressive neuropathy	10
Splenomegaly	9
Episcleritis	9
Pericarditis	2

Adopted from Gordon, Stein, and Broder. Am J Med 54:445–452, 1973.

patients with RA. Usually they are located on the extensor surface of the forearms in the region of the olecranon bursa or more distally. The nodules are firm, nontender, oval or rounded masses that vary in size from 0.5 to 2 cm. Although generally freely movable, they may become fixed to the underlying periosteum. Less commonly, they are found on the Achilles tendon, occiput, or ischial tuberosities, in synovial and periarticular tissues, and in internal organs (e.g., heart, intestinal tract). Rarely seen in early disease, they are usually associated with active synovitis, positive serum rheumatoid factor (RF), and a poor prognosis. The histologic features of rheumatoid nodules include an irregularly shaped central zone of fibrinoid necrosis surrounded by large mononuclear cells (chiefly macrophages) that are palisaded around the central necrotic area, an outer zone of granulation tissue containing lymphocytes and plasma cells, and a surrounding area of fibrous tissue.

Subclinical cardiac disease is frequent in RA, being found in 50% of patients by echocardiographic and other techniques and at autopsy (Table 4). Patients with symptomatic pericarditis usually are RF positive (95%) and have subcutaneous rheumatoid nodules (45%). Left anterior chest pain (60%) and pericardial friction rub (65%) are present commonly. Cardiomegaly is almost invariably found, and pleural effusions (65%) and clinical findings of congestive heart failure (20%) are often evident. The pericardial fluid contains between 1000 and 28,000/mm^3 WBC, 5–10 g/dl protein, elevated gamma globulin and cholesterol levels, and depressed glucose and total hemolytic complement concentrations. Immune complexes and RF are detected at times.

TABLE 4
Cardiac Involvement in RA

Chronic Pericarditis	50% (autopsy)
Echocardiographic abnormalities (thickening and/or effusion)	47%
Mitral valve abnormalities	30% (slowing)
Coronary arteritis	20% (autopsy)
Aortitis, dilatation of aortic root	
Rheumatoid nodules	
Lethal arrhythmias	

Cardiac tamponade and constrictive pericarditis are unusual but life-threatening complications of RA that require surgical intervention. Results from systemic corticosteroid treatment and pericardiocentesis are unsatisfactory, as the pericardial fluid generally is thick and loculated.

The pleura and/or pulmonary parenchyma may be affected by RA; the spectrum of lung disease is shown in Table 5. Pleural effusions are characterized by low glucose concentrations (usually less than 10 mg/dl and are attributed to a disturbed sugar transport mechanism across the pleural membrane), a diminution in whole hemolytic complement and complement components (suggesting a local immunologic reaction), numerous large multinucleated cells, a positive RF, and a markedly elevated lactic dehydrogenase.

Caplan's syndrome occurs primarily in Welsh coal miners, but it may affect any RA patient who is chronically exposed to siliceous dusts. Multiple well-defined nodular opacities 0.5 to 5 cm in diameter are distributed throughout the lungs, but particularly peripherally. Histologically, the lesions are rheumatoid granulomas. There may be little or no roentgenographic evidence of pneumoconiosis, and the nodules may appear before, coincident with, or after the onset of arthritis. Serum RF generally is strongly positive.

There are numerous eye findings in RA including keratoconjunctivitis sicca, episcleritis, keratitis, iridocyclitis, scleromalacia, and scleromalacia perforans. Eye problems tend to be bilateral and generally are associated with subcutaneous nodules, vasculitis, and other systemic manifestations. Rheumatoid granulomas may be found on the sclera.

TABLE 5
Pulmonary Involvement in RA

Diffuse interstitial fibrosis	~ 1%
Pleural effusion	~ 3%
Rheumatoid nodules (subpleural, intraparenchymal)	
Cavitary lesions	
Caplan's syndrome	
Pleural adhesions	40% (autopsy)
History of pleurisy	20%
Abnormal pulmonary function tests	47% (↓ gas transfer)

TABLE 6
Neurologic Manifestations of RA

I. Articular: Cervical spine disease
  A. Cervical subluxations
    1. C_1 moves anteriorly on C_2
    2. C_1 moves posteriorly on C_2
    3. Vertical subluxation of odontoid
    4. Multiple lower level subluxations
  B. Narrowed disc spaces
  C. Asymptomatic radiologic findings: Vertebral plate and apophyseal joint erosions, basilar impression of the skull

II. Extraarticular
  A. Peripheral neuropathies
    1. Entrapment
    2. Mild sensory
    3. Diffuse sensorimotor
    4. Fulminant sensorimotor
  B. Vasculitis
    1. Mononeuritis complex
    2. Cerebral vasculitis
  C. Dural rheumatoid nodules: brain, spinal cord compression

Rheumatoid arthritis may also be associated with a variety of neurologic difficulties, especially nerve compression syndromes, less frequently with a chronic sensory polyneuropathy, and uncommonly with an acute, severe sensorimotor neuropathy (mononeuritis multiplex) (Table 6). The last named is found with other evidence of systemic vasculitis and appears to be the result of a necrotizing angiitis of the vasa nervorum. It is characterized by deposition of IgG, IgM, and complement components in blood vessel walls.

A variety of skin lesions have been described on RA patients (Table 7). Ischemic skin ulcers, especially of the distal leg near the malleoli,

TABLE 7
Skin Involvement in RA

Subcutaneous rheumatoid nodules	Livedo reticularis
Raynaud's phenomenon	Ulcers
Digital infarcts	Cutaneous atrophy
Peripheral gangrene	Palmar erythema
Purpuric papules; hemorrhagic bullae	

digital infarcts, and peripheral gangrene generally are found in chronic seropositive disease and more frequently in Felty's syndrome. These lesions result from arteritis and may or may not respond to vigorous medical and surgical management.

Anemia, often normocytic and normo- or hypochromic, is the most frequent hematologic abnormality noted; the magnitude of anemia generally correlates with rheumatoid activity. Iron absorption is normal and slightly decreased, bone marrow iron reserves usually are normal, but synovial iron content is markedly increased. Plasma volume may be increased slightly causing a hemodilution effect, but bone marrow red cell production is not increased. Leukopenia, leukocytosis, and eosinophilia occur uncommonly. Splenomegaly may be an isolated finding or may be found in association with Felty's syndrome.

Secondary amyloidosis occurs in approximately 10% of cases, but the prevalence of this disorder varies widely from series to series (5–61%). Postmortem versus in vivo studies, different patient populations, and diverse techniques used to define amyloid deposits are causes for this variability.

Avascular necrosis of one or both femoral heads or, less commonly, other bones may develop, frequently in association with corticosteroid treatment. Osteoporosis, related to corticosteroid therapy, disuse, or other effects of RA, may lead to spontaneous fractures of vertebrae or long bones.

LABORATORY TESTS

Numerous specific laboratory abnormalities are found in RA patients, the majority of which are listed here.

Blood Elements

Erythrocyte—moderate normochromic or hypochromic, normocytic anemia; low plasma iron; moderately decreased marrow iron stores; normal utilization of plasma iron; slightly decreased erythrocyte survival time; inadequate release of iron from tissue stores.

Leukocytes—normal or slightly elevated in most adult cases; leukopenia rare; eosinophilia occasional; leukocytosis with left shift common in juvenile disease.

Acute Phase Phenomena

Erythrocyte sedimentation rate (ESR)—moderately to markedly increased in most patients.

C-reactive protein—present in majority; parallels the ESR.

Serum protein—alpha-2 globulin, fibrinogen, and gamma globulin usually increased; alpha-1 globulin may be increased; albumin usually decreased and beta globulin unchanged.

Seromucoid, protein-bound hexose, and haptoglobin—usually increased.

Mucopolysaccharide excretion—usually elevated in adults and decreased in children.

Immune Factors

LE cell—present in about 10%.

ANA—present in 25-50%.

RF—present in majority of adult cases (about 75%).

Biologic false-positive (BFP) serology reaction—present in 5-10%.

Complement—usually normal or somewhat elevated.

Immunoconglutinin—usually elevated.

Liver Function

Alkaline phosphatase, SGOT, and SGPT—occasionally slightly elevated.

Renal Function

Proteinuria—may be present due to amyloidosis, unrelated renal disease, or medication (e.g. gold compounds, penicillamine).

Creatinine clearance—often shows some decrease.

Miscellaneous

3-hydroxyanthranilic acid and kynurenine excretion—often increased.

Blood cholesterol—often reduced.

Blood vitamin levels—usually decreased.

Serum ceruloplasmin and serum copper—usually elevated.

Gastric acidity—often reduced in patients under 40.

Synovial fluid changes are given in Table 1 of the previous chapter on Synovianalysis.

TREATMENT

Treatment is dependent upon many factors including the severity and extent of the disease process; the degree of disability; the presence or absence of extraarticular manifestations, bone erosions, joint space narrowing, and deformity; the results of previous treatment; and numerous social, psychologic, and economic variables (8). At the onset, conservative measures used most frequently include moderate to high doses of salicylates, periods of rest, splints, and instructions regarding activities of daily living. For those patients who fail to respond to this regimen, additional stronger analgesic or antiinflammatory medications may be necessary. Indomethacin (Indocin), usually in doses of 75-100 mg daily, is helpful in some patients. Newer nonsteroidal antiinflammatory agents include ibuprofen (Motrin), naproxen (Naprosyn), tolmetin (Tolectin), fenoprofen (Nalfon), and sulindac (Clinoril). All these compounds possess analgesic and antiinflammatory properties and cause fewer gastrointestinal symptoms and less G.I. bleeding, tinnitus, dizziness, and light-headedness than salicylates. They equal but do not exceed salicylates in efficacy.

For patients with persistent articular complaints, chloroquine or hydroxychloroquine may be added to the regimen. Treatment of several months is usually necessary before improvement occurs. Dermatitis and gastrointestinal distress are the most frequently noted side effects, but these are not as potentially serious as the occasional visual disturbance that develops. Drug accumulation in the cornea may be associated with dimness of vision or halo formation. This kerotapathy is fully reversible with cessation of therapy. However, antimalarials preferentially deposit in the pigment layer of the retina, leading to degenerative changes that result in progressive visual loss that may advance despite abandonment of therapy. Complete ophthalmologic examination should be performed prior to initiation of treatment and at 3- to 6-month intervals thereafter.

Chrysotherapy (gold compounds) is used for uncontrolled active RA—especially when joint deformities, juxtaarticular osseous erosions, or extraarticular disease develops—with favorable results in the majority of patients (9). Improvement seldom occurs until several months after initiation of therapy. Following test doses, 50 mg of aurothioglucose (Solganal) or gold sodium thiomalate (Myochrysine) is administered intramuscularly on a weekly basis until 1 g is reached or until improvement or toxicity develops. Subsequently, maintenance gold therapy consisting of 50 mg every 2 to 4 weeks is recommended. The most frequent side effects are dermatitis and stomatitis. Other more serious but less common complications of chrysotherapy include bone marrow depression and renal damage, necessitating frequent blood counts and urine analyses throughout treatment. An orally administered gold preparation (Auranofin) triethylphosphine gold is undergoing intensive clinical testing but is not yet commercially available.

Intraarticular corticosteroids are helpful in relieving symptoms and decreasing joint inflammation. Because of possible deleterious effects on cartilage, repeated injections into the same joint generally should not be given more often than every 2 months. Careful monitoring is mandatory.

Although systemic corticosteroids are used to treat active RA, and often dramatically alleviate pain and stiffness, chronic administration is associated with numerous undesirable side effects. If corticosteroids are used, low dosages should be given (e.g., 10 mg or less daily of prednisone) or they should be administered on an alternate day schedule. If severe extraarticular manifestations of RA are present (e.g., vasculitis), aggressive therapy, sometimes in the range of 60 to 100 mg of prednisone daily, may be warranted.

Histidine, an amino acid, has been used based in part on the findings of low serum histidine levels in RA, which return to normal during recovery. Although its therapeutic efficacy is not established in controlled double-blind studies, side effects are minimal. Histidine is administered orally, 4 to 6 g daily.

D-penicillamine (Cuprimine, Depen) also suppresses rheumatoid synovitis, although its mechanisms of action are largely unknown (10). Serum rheumatoid factor, immunoglobulin concentrations, and the erythrocyte sedimentation rate are reduced. Rheumatoid subcutaneous nodules may diminish in size or disappear, and vasculitis may be controlled. D-penicillamine and gold compounds appear equally effective in double-blind studies. The frequency of adverse reactions to D-penicillamine, and the occasional severe reaction (thrombocytopenia, aplastic anemia, nephrotic syndrome, and a variety of autoimmune disorders), mandates careful monitoring by clinicians skilled in its use and fully aware of its side effects.

Cytotoxic agents are not approved by the FDA for the treatment of RA. Cyclophosphamide (Cytoxan), azathioprine (Imuran), methotrexate, and other similar drugs reduce the symptoms and signs of inflammatory joint disease and in some cases retard cartilage and bone destruction. Because of multiple side effects including bone marrow depression, enhanced susceptibility to infection, liver dysfunction, and lymphoid tumor induction, these agents are reserved primarily for patients with unusually disabling disease who have failed to respond to more conservative measures.

Levamisole, an oral antihelminthic agent with immunostimulatory properties, is another experimental agent of value in RA (11). Serious untoward effects, especially hematopoeitic (e.g., agranulocytosis), have stimulated controlled studies using lower dosage schedules. The proper place for this agent in the therapeutic armamentarium is speculative.

Medical synovectomy, using radioactive colloidal gold or yttrium, or chemical synovectomy using osmium tetroxide (osmic acid), has been used for several decades in Europe to treat severely inflamed large joints. These agents are particularly effective in treating joints subject to recurrent large effusions. This therapeutic modality has received only limited attention in the United States for several reasons, including systemic leakage from the intraarticular space, chromosomal damage, possible carcinogenic effects, and possibly injury to the articular cartilage.

The use of "early" or "prophylactic" surgical synovectomy in RA remains controversial, although ample evidence shows regrowth of inflamed tissues in most patients. Generally, the duration of improvement following synovectomy is 3 to 5 years.

Reconstructive orthopedic surgery (see the closing chapter on Total Joint Replacement) for patients with severe deforming arthritis, poorly controlled pain, or significant functional disability is more widely advocated than previously, in part due to technical advances in materials and methods. Silastic prostheses for joints of the wrist, hand, and foot and total hip and knee joint replacement often afford dramatic benefit to patients who otherwise would have remained incapacitated.

REFERENCES

1. Short CL, Bauer W, Reynolds WE, Rheumatoid Arthritis. Cambridge, MA: Harvard University Press, 1957.
2. Williams RC Jr. Clinical picture of rheumatoid arthritis. In: McCarty DJ, ed. Arthritis and Allied Conditions. Philadelphia: Lea & Febiger, 1979, 9th ed., p. 457.
3. Harris ED Jr. Pathogenesis of rheumatoid arthritis. In: Kelley WN, Har-

ris ED Jr, Ruddy S, Sledge CS, eds. Textbook of Rheumatology. Philadelphia: Saunders, 1981, p. 896.

4. Gray RG, Gottlieb, NL. Hand flexor tenosynovitis in rheumatoid arthritis. Arthritis Rheum 20:1003-1008, 1977.
5. Hurd ER. Extra-articular manifestations of rheumatoid arthritis. Semin Arthritis Rheum 8:151-176, 1979.
6. Hart FD. Extra-articular manifestations of rheumatoid arthritis. Semin Arthritis Rheum 1:161-173, 1971.
7. Gordon DA, Stein JL, Broder I. The extra-articular features of rheumatoid arthritis. Am J Med 54:445-452, 1973.
8. Ruddy SH. The management of rheumatoid arthritis. In: Kelley WN, Harris ED Jr, Ruddy S, Sledge CB, eds. Textbook of Rheumatology. Philadelphia: Saunders, 1981, p. 1000.
9. Gottlieb, NL. Chrysotherapy. Bull Rheum Dis 27:912-913, 1976-77.
10. Jaffee IA. D-penicillamine. Bull Rheum Dis 28:948-952, 1977-78.
11. International symposium on levamisole in rheumatoid arthritis. J Rheumatol 5 (Suppl 4):1-2, 1978.

JUVENILE RHEUMATOID ARTHRITIS

WILBUR J. BLECHMAN, M.D.

Stillman and Barry described juvenile rheumatoid arthritis (JRA) as "an ill-defined rheumatic disease beginning before the sixteenth birthday" (1). Schaller in the same journal noted that while JRA patients "share the common characteristic of chronic synovitis," it is doubtful that JRA is a single disease (2).

In spite of these apparent differences, each observer, as well as a number of others, separate JRA into specific arbitrarily defined subgroups (3). The classification most often used depends on the mode of onset and is endowed with certain prognostic implications as follows:

1. Systemic
2. Pauciarticular—defined as four or fewer joints
3. Polyarticular—defined as more than four joints

It is estimated that more than 250,000 children in the United States are afflicted.

PRESENTATIONS

Systemic disease onset has been observed in approximately 20% of JRA patients. These children are febrile, usually with temperatures above 101° F. Fever may be 106° F or higher. A typical, salmon-colored macular rash may be present, especially during febrile periods. It may fade and disappear as the temperature falls. Rash is most common centrally and can be induced by slight trauma (Koebner phenomenon), which may be helpful in suggesting the diagnosis.

Lymphadenopathy (sometimes marked), hepatosplenomegaly, pleuritis, and/or pericarditis may be found in this group. The systemic form shares with the polyarticular group a 50% incidence of involvement of the cervical spine. Other joints are variably affected both in incidence and severity and may follow the onset of fever by weeks or months (Fig. 1). Calabro has reported cases that have never developed a true synovitis; nevertheless they show all or most of the features of systemic onset JRA (4).

Approximately 66% of systemic onset patients develop their disease before the age of 5. Sex incidence is equal in this group. Incidence is higher for girls in the other age groups. Systemic symptoms, as just described, may be associated with anemia, leukocytosis, and a high sedimentation rate and may persist for as long as 6 consecutive months. Schaller has reported recurrence of this systemic disease symptom complex in 50% of 22 patients (2).

The arthritis that develops with systemic onset responds to proper therapy in the majority of cases. However, 25% will experience severe arthritis followed by demonstrable disability. Pauciarticular onset oc-

FIGURE 1
Extensive erosions of elbow joint.

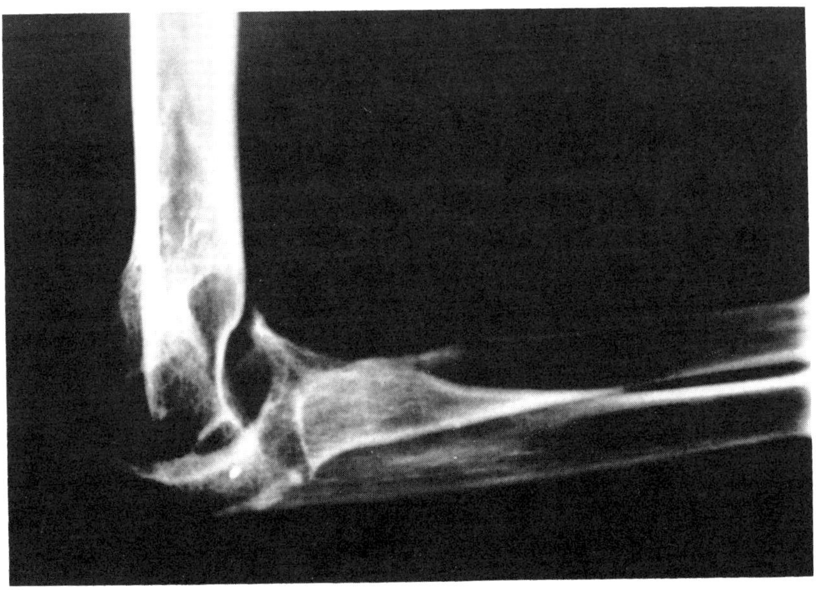

curs in 33% of the cases. The knee and ankle are the joints most commonly involved (Fig. 2). This type occurs primarily in girls, usually developing before 5 years of age. This group has the least morbidity and best prognosis of all JRA subgroups. A high incidence of iridocyclitis is a critical complication. This is usually insidious in development. It frequently leads to visual loss or blindness when undiagnosed and untreated.

Approximately 90% of children with JRA and chronic iridocyclitis have positive tests for antinuclear antibodies (ANA) (2). Thus ANA is accepted as a marker for this group of patients at special risk for

FIGURE 2
Narrowing of joint space and chronic synovitis of knee.

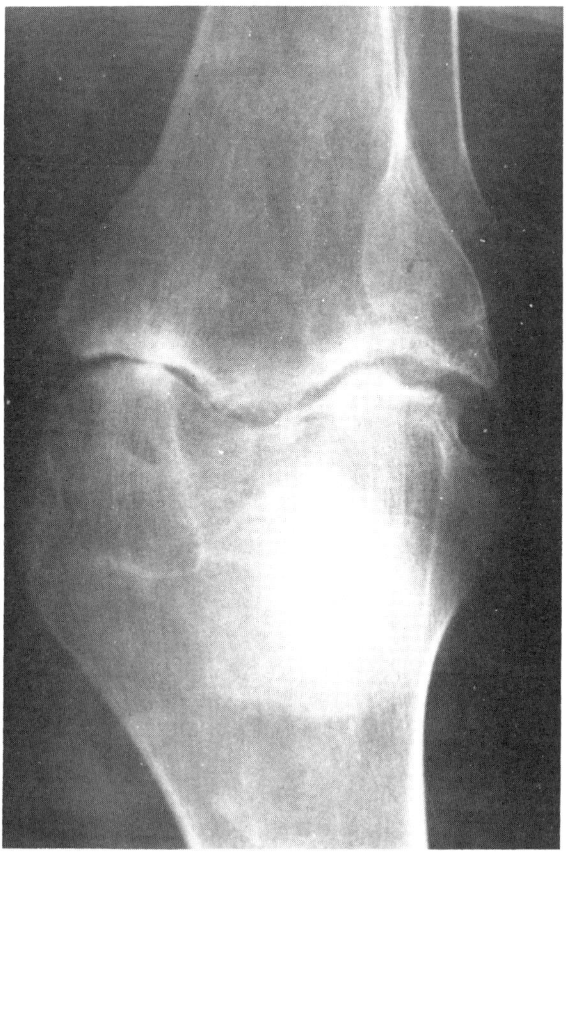

blindness. Ansell suggests that the ANA positive group of pauciarticular children receive slit-lamp examination every 4 months (5). Lack of ANA is no guarantee that the patient will not develop chronic iridocyclitis, althought the risk seems much less. Yearly slit-lamp evaluation is recommended for those in the ANA-negative group.

It has been recognized in recent years that previous studies of JRA have included children destined to develop ankylosing spondylitis but with a pauciarticular onset of peripheral joint disease (Fig. 3). This group, mainly male and with symptoms beginning at a later age, are

FIGURE 3

X-ray of hand showing extensive changes in bones and joints; several are similar to findings in adult rheumatoid arthritis.

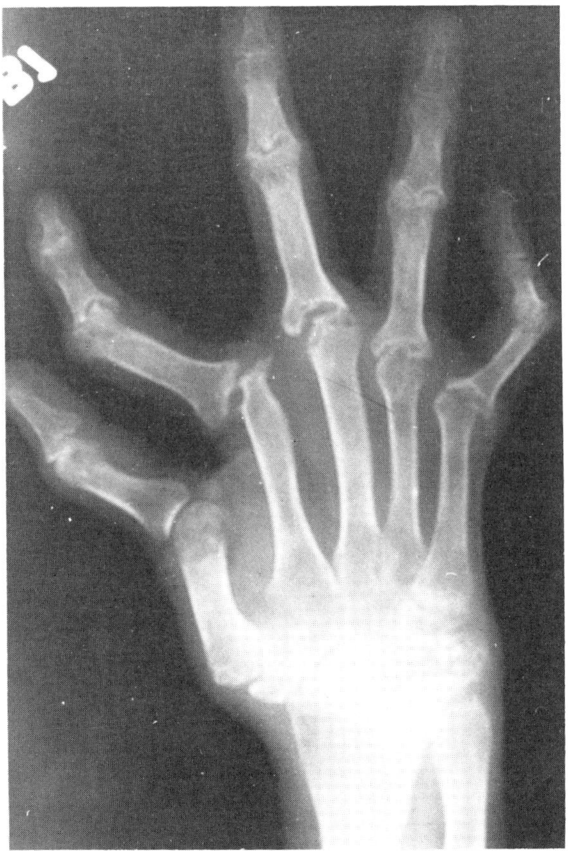

more susceptible to hip involvement with a positive HLA-B27 antigen. These children should be classified as having ankylosing spondylitis rather than JRA. The correct diagnosis may not be apparent for some time.

The most common mode of onset is polyarticular. This is characteristic of approximately 50% of patients. It is twice as frequent in girls. Large joints are frequently involved as are those of the hands and feet. Cervical spine involvement, as with the systemic onset, is common and is suggested by a loss of neck extension (Fig. 4). This form of presentation occurs at all ages but is more common after the age of 10. Systemic symptoms are more likely to occur than in the pauciarticular subset but are less common and less marked than with

FIGURE 4
Marked micrognathia in a patient with progressive cervical involvement.

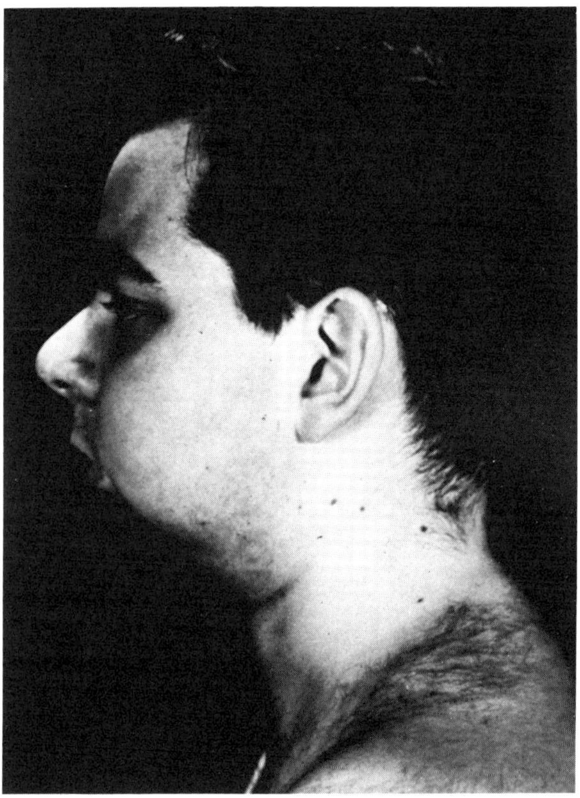

the systemic disease onset. Although the sedimentation rate may be elevated, rheumatoid factor usually is absent. If rheumatoid factor is positive, it is most probable that the condition is adult rheumatoid arthritis appearing at a younger age than usual. Polyarticular disease has a poorer functional prognosis than the other subsets. This is most pronounced when the disease begins in the early years of life. Polyarticular, rheumatoid factor-positive JRA has the poorest prognosis with eventual joint destruction and disability.

DIAGNOSIS

No attempt will be made to present a complete differential of all possible diagnoses. It is evident that the same arthritides that affect adults may also affect children. Special emphasis should be placed on such possibilities as acute rheumatic fever, infectious arthritis, trauma (e.g., battered child syndrome), and such hematologic disorders as hemophilia, sickle cell disease, and leukemia. Any of these may initially be confusing. Time and the clinical course of the disease are the physician's best allies in establishing the correct diagnosis.

THERAPY

The social, psychologic, and educational needs of the child as well as medical therapy must be considered in all subgroups of JRA. Parents must be involved and should be informed of many of the critical aspects of the disease and how it is likely to affect their child as well as their relationships with the child. Every attempt should be made to allow the child to live as normal a life as possible, recognizing that certain compromises in activity are needed to prevent harm to the joints. Each child must be evaluated and treated according to the individual needs. Specific exercises, physical therapy, and mechanical aids should be reviewed when indicated and should be started under the guidance of a qualified physical and/or occupational therapist.

Medical therapy for all forms usually is helpful. The mainstay of treatment is aspirin in doses beginning with 100 mg/Kg of body weight per day, given in four to six divided doses. Cases intolerant of aspirin or other salicylates may respond to Tolmetin. For unresponsive JRA, gold therapy or D-penicillamine has been helpful. As previously noted, slit-lamp examination is indicated yearly in pauciarticular (and possibly polyarticular as well) onset, even if the arthritis remits. If ANA are present in either pauci- or polyarticular disease, this examination should be performed every 4 months in case of incipient potentially blinding iridocyclitis. When found this should be treated by the ophthalmologist. It may require local or systemic corticosteroids.

Except for the ophthalmologic use of corticosteroids, these compounds are rarely indicated. The risks of corticosteroid therapy in JRA seem excessive for whatever potential value they may offer.

REFERENCES

1. Stillman JS, Barry PE. Juvenile rheumatoid arthritis: series 2. Arthritis Rheum 20(Suppl):171-175, 1977.
2. Schaller JG. Juvenile rheumatoid arthritis: series 1. Arthritis Rheum 20(Suppl):165-169, 1977.
3. Brewer EJ, Bass J, Baum J, et al. Current proposed revision of JRA criteria. Arthritis Rheum 20(Suppl):195-199, 1977.
4. Calabro JJ, Burnstein SL, Staley HL. JRA posing as fever of unknown origin. Arthritis Rheum 20(Suppl):178-180, 1977.
5. Ansell BM. Chronic arthritis in childhood. Ann Rheum Dis 37:107-120, 1978.

ANKYLOSING SPONDYLITIS

HARVEY E. BROWN, M.D.

Ankylosing spondylitis (AS) is a chronic, progressive form of arthritis distinct from RA (1). Ankylosis of a number of joints, involving primarily the spine and paraspinal structures, is the usual end result. The cause is unknown. Males are affected 4:1. The disease is characterized by nonfebrile inflammation of the sacroiliac joints (Fig. 1), the spinal apophyseal joints (Fig. 2), and the paravertebral soft tissue. Ossification of the annulus fibrosus of the intervertebral discs and of the connective tissue immediately adjacent to the annulus and alterations in the intervertebral diarthrodial joints eventually lead to fibrosis.

CLINICAL FINDINGS

The disease usually appears in the second or third decade of life. The family incidence is high; frequently two or more close relatives may be afflicted. There is a predominant incidence of the histocompatibility antigen HLA-B27, as well as a lower but significant incidence in nonaffected relatives (2).

The beginning of the disease is insidious with little more than a low backache in the sacroiliac joints or over the hips. There may be sciatic radiation. Morning stiffness of the back muscles is the counterpart of morning stiffness of the hands in RA. Symptoms tend to progress. With involvement of the dorsal and lumbar spine, motion of the back and expansion of the chest is restricted. Eventually, the symphysis pubis and manubriosternal joints are affected as well as the shoulders and sometimes the knees (Fig. 3) and other more peripheral joints.

Constitutional symptoms, which include fever, fatigue, and weight

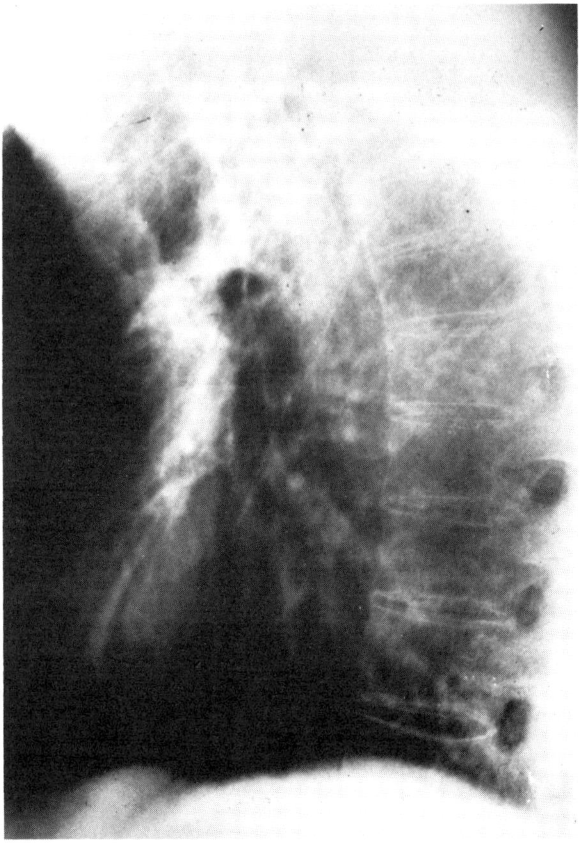

FIGURE 1
Extensive involvement of sacroiliac joints and lumbar spine.

loss, are usually mild. Iritis or iridocyclitis may precede joint symptoms but rarely causes serious eye trouble. Cardiac conduction may be impaired with first degree AV block. There may be an associated aortic insufficiency, which increases in probability with the duration of the disease and the degree of peripheral joint involvement. Neither subcutaneous nodules nor the visceral lesions of RA develop.

Examination of the sacroiliac joints usually shows tenderness on palpation or limitation of motion when the legs are flexed on the abdomen; straightening of the normal lumbar lordosis may follow with immobility of the lumbar spine on forward bending and spasm

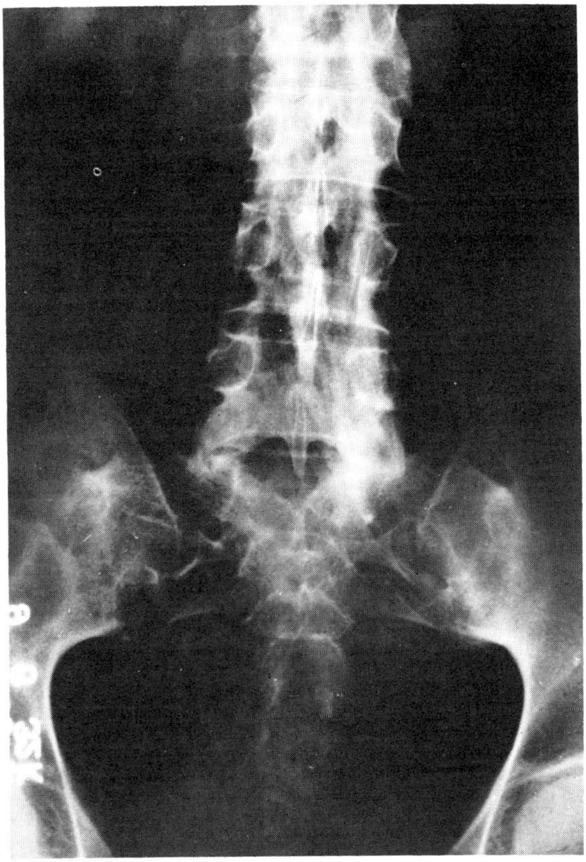

FIGURE 2
Squaring of vertebral bodies with syndesmophyte formation.

of the paravertebral muscles. In the late stages, the entire spine, from the first cervical vertebra to the sacroiliac articulation, may be fixed and immobile. Either a "poker spine" in the erect position or a hump back or dorsal kyphosis with forward flexion of the thoracic spine is the result. Neck movements may be limited. Expansion of the chest is restricted with a decrease in vital capacity and with flattening of the anterior thoracic cage and involvement of the costovertebral joints. Apical pulmonary fibrosis has been described.

The findings on microscopic examination are essentially those of adult RA with chronic proliferative synovitis. Later, fibrosis of the

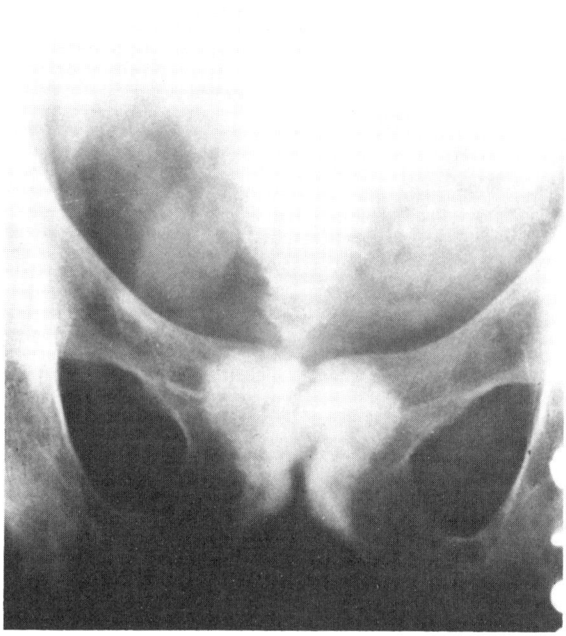

FIGURE 3
Arthritis of symphysis pubis in ankylosing spondylitis.

capsule and bony ankylosis of the joints, ossification of the interspinous ligaments and the capsular ligaments of the vertebral apophyseal joints, and the formation of bony bridges, syndesmophytes, unite the lateral and internal margins of adjacent vertebrae. Amyloidosis has been reported at necropsy in 5% of patients.

LABORATORY FINDINGS

The erythrocyte sedimentation rate may be normal. A mild anemia may be present. The incidence of RF is low. HLA B27 is present in 90% of cases.

The x-ray findings are almost pathognomonic. The earliest change in the sacroiliac joints, on one or both sides, is blurring of the subchondral bony margins. Erosions develop particularly on the iliac side and are associated with patchy sclerosis on both sides of the articulations with narrowing of the interosseous joint space. Eventually, the sacroiliacs become fused and syndesmophytes bridge adjacent vertebrae. In advanced cases the ossification of syndesmophytes of the vertebrae are responsible for the appearance of what has been identified as a "bamboo spine." The bodies of the vertebrae tend to assume a square contour that is especially evident in the lateral projection. In some patients the vertebral bodies may show varying degrees of bony demineralization with a ballooning appearance of the intervertebral discs (Figure 1). There may be subluxation of the atlantoaxial vertebrae in the cervical spine.

CLINICAL COURSE

The disease is progressive, advancing from the sacroiliacs cephalad. It is unpredictable in the individual case. From 10 to 20 years may be required for the development of a poker spine or cervicodorsal kyphosis. A small percentage of patients become arthritic cripples.

THERAPY

Aspirin remains the drug of choice, combined with physical therapy. Stronger drugs such as phenylbutazone (100 to 200 mg/day) or indomethacin (100 to 150 mg/day) may be helpful. Either of these drugs for long periods of time should be avoided because of the incidence of side effects. Muscle relaxants are not effective. Resort to corticosteroids is rarely necessary. Gold is not helpful. X-ray therapy to the spine is contraindicated. Iritis should be treated in consultation with an ophthalmologist; corticosteroids are recommended for this complication.

The importance of postural exercises and heat, which should be carried out several times a day, should be appreciated. The erect position should be maintained when standing or sitting. Flexion postures should be kept at a minimum. Breathing exercises should be taught early, and upper respiratory infection should be controlled. Scheduled rest periods during the day may be helpful. The mattress for sleeping should be firm, probably supported by bed boards. The supine position is almost obligatory with a minimum of time in the flexed position. The head should not be elevated with a pillow. Splints or molds provide proper positioning of joints threatened by ankylosis. A back brace may be supportive in advanced disease. Various surgical procedures including the hips may be indicated.

REFERENCES

1. Sigler JW. Clinical features of ankylosing spondylitis. Clin Orthop 74:41-49, 1971.
2. Brewerton DA, James DCO. The histocompatibility antigen (HL-A 27) and disease. Semin Arthritis Rheum 4:191-207, 1975.

PSORIATIC ARTHRITIS

DAVID S. HOWELL, M.D.

CLINICAL CHARACTERISTICS

There is a highly significant association of the skin lesions of psoriasis and polyarthritis with different types of presentation of joint disease (1). The most common form is peripheral asymmetric polyarthritis involving, among many sites, most frequently the distal interphalangeal joints. A second type is a destructive form, arthritis mutilans (Fig. 1), with a similar distribution to the previous type and, in addition, a high frequency of spondylitis (2). A third clinical type, rarely seen, is rheumatoid arthritic coincident with psoriasis, indistinguishable in every respect.

The distal interphalangeal, proximal interphalangeal, and metacarpophalangeal joints of the hands and metatarsophalangeal joints of the feet are the commonest sites of involvement. Gradually, over the years, there develop bulbous deformities and diffuse, cylindrical thickening of the digits called sausage fingers or toes (Fig. 2), features that help distinguish the disease from classic rheumatoid arthritis. Inflammatory activity tends to vary with the skin disease although there are exceptions. The course of the disease in general is less severe than that of rheumatoid arthritis. In about 75% of the psoriatic patients with arthritis the nails of the hands and/or feet are involved, whereas nail involvement is found in about only 30% of patients lacking arthritis. There is frequently disease in the distal phalanges adjacent to thickened, pitted nails. All psoriatic patients are prone to involvement of the spine and sacroiliac joints. When this occurs, syndesmophytes tend to arise from the lateral and anterior surfaces of vertebral bodies (Fig. 3). Conjunctivitis and iritis may occur.

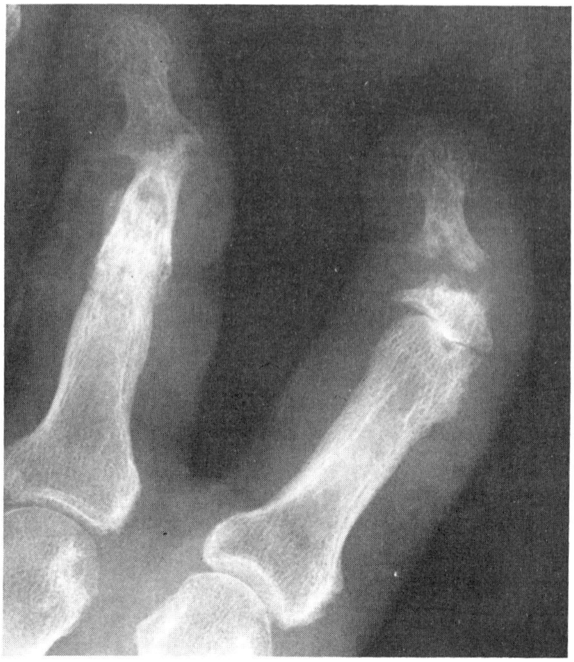

FIGURE 1
Radiologic changes in the digits in psoriatic arthritis.

An important distinctive feature is the presence of a position histocompatibility laboratory test (HLA-B27) with the blood cells of patients with psoriasis, as well as the absence of rheumatoid factor and absence of subcutaneous nodules (3). There are also less specific changes such as elevated sedimentation rate, mild anemia, and elevated alpha-2 globulin. Serum uric acid levels may be increased and lead to a false diagnosis of gouty arthritis, especially where there are objective changes in the great toe of heat, redness, and swelling. The elevated uric acid is believed to result from a rapid purine turnover in inflamed skin.

Radiologic features of psoriatic arthritis are variable. On the one extreme, there may be only mild local osteoporosis in juxtaarticular bone. At the other extreme, there may be large punched-out lesions adjacent to joints, particularly in the digits. A pencil-and-cup deformity of whittling of terminal phalanges and osteolysis are seen particularly in arthritis mutilans. Fluffy margins of the bone are consis-

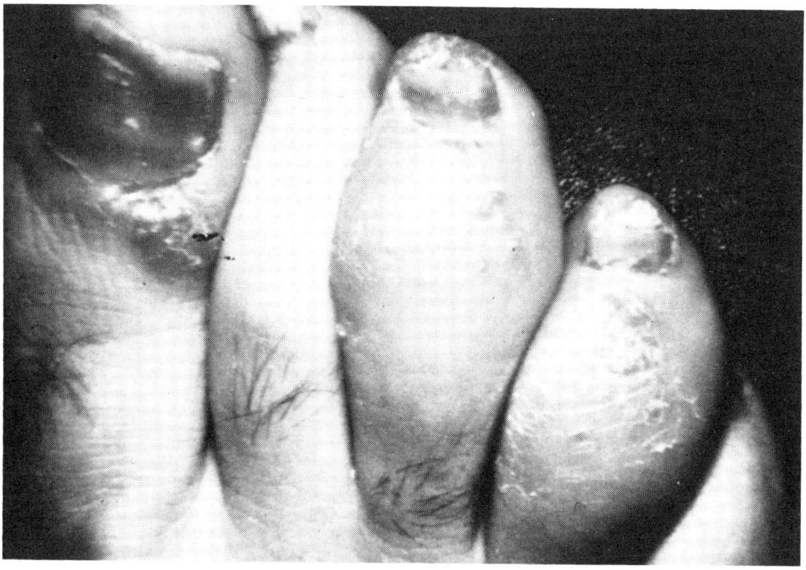

FIGURE 2
Sausage toes and psoriatic lesions of skin and nails

tent with periostitis, as on the calcaneus, and in the spine the syndesmophytes arise not only at the margins but back a centimeter or so from the edges of the vertebrae.

Dramatic responses to treatment are uncommon. If only mild to moderate disease is present, relief of joint pain and stiffness may be obtained with buffered aspirin or other antiinflammatory drugs such as ibuprofen, indomethacin, or phenylbutazone, along with the conventional measures for cutaneous disease. Often, moderate response in most of the joints is obtained, but if a small number of joints are still severely painful, local corticosteroid injections are helpful temporarily. In severe disease unresponsive to these measures immunosuppressive drugs such as azathioprine (Imuran) may be tried cautiously. Methotrexate causes such serious liver damage that only a few of the severest cases should be considered for this treatment. Chrysotherapy has been discouraged although adequate study of this form of management is lacking. Hydroxychloroquine (Plaquenil) and chloroquine are believed to aggravate the skin disease.

Reconstructive surgery and arthrodesis are helpful in selected situations where cartilage damage and joint instability have ensued.

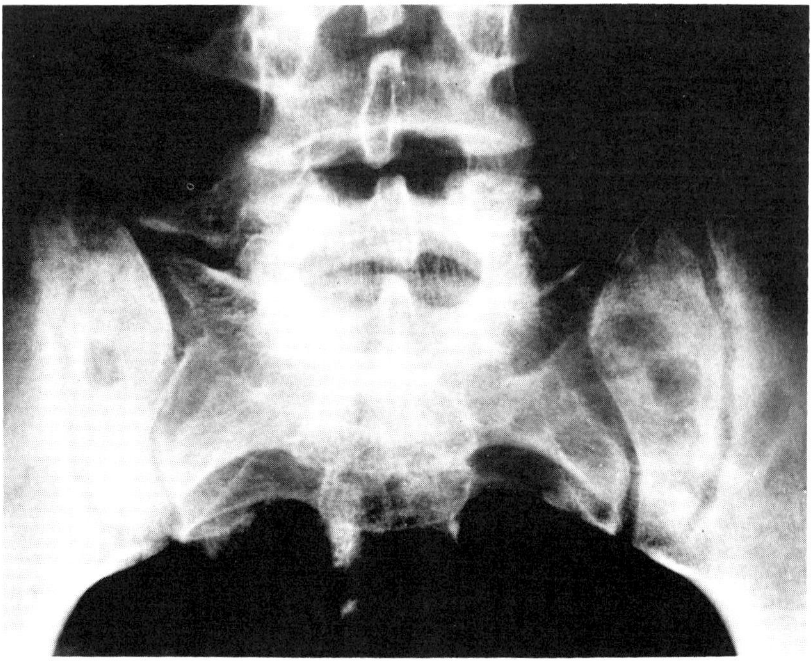

FIGURE 3
Sacroiliitis in psoriatic arthritis.

Synovectomy has not proved to have more than temporary value in relief of acute boggy knees or other joints due to rapid regrowth of the inflamed synovium.

REFERENCES

1. Moll JMH, Wright V. Psoriatic arthritis. Semin Arthritis Rheum 3:55-78, 1973.
2. McEwen C, Di Tata D, Lingg C. Ankylosing spondylitis and spondylitis accompanying ulcerative colitis, regional enteritis, psoriasis, and Reiter's disease: a comparative study. Arthritis Rheum 14:291-318, 1971.
3. Gray RG, Gottlieb NL. The HL-A B27 histocompatibility antigen in rheumatoid arthritis. J Fla Med Assoc 63:339-344, 1976.
4. Lambert JR, Wright V. Eye inflammation in psoriatic arthritis. Ann Rheum Dis 35:354-356, 1976.

FELTY'S SYNDROME

DAVID S. HOWELL, M.D.

Felty's syndrome is considered a variant of rheumatoid arthritis, appearing in 4 to 5% of patients (1,2). The syndrome consists of deforming arthritis, splenomegaly, and leukopenia. In addition, patients may show weight loss and pigmentation on exposed surfaces of skin. The arthritis usually begins a decade or more before the onset of splenomegaly. Most patients present with this syndrome in the fifth to seventh decade. The rheumatoid disease is usually manifested by irreversible deformities, subcutaneous nodules, and rheumatoid factor in high titer.

The spleen may be barely palpable or extremely large and tender. Chronic ulcerations of the legs overlying the ankles and lower tibial regions are common. These ulcers may be painful, deeply ulcerated, and usually contain a mixed flora. There is often vascular impairment involving both the arterial and venous systems. Other associated clinical manifestations of peripheral neuropathy, episcleritis, and pericarditis are present less commonly.

Laboratory studies may show a leukocyte count ranging from 1000 to 4300/mm^3, with differential counts showing a preponderant reduction in neutrophil leukocytes. There is hypochromic anemia typical of rheumatoid arthritis. Studies on red cell survival indicate accelerated production and destruction of marrow cells. The reserve of granulocytes after an etiocholanolone test for granulocyte reserve shows a reduction of cells liberated from reserve sites. Depressed leucocyte function has been demonstrated together with an abnormal leucocyte uptake of immunoglobulins.

Because of a high incidence of antinuclear factor positivity and presence of LE cell positivity in some patients, an overlap with systemic lupus erythematosus has been proposed. However, the absence of disease in the central nervous system and kidneys makes uncertain a relationship to SLE.

Treatment includes the usual conservative regimen for rheumatoid arthritis. In addition, patients suffering from recurrent infection, not cured by local antibiotics and hygienic measures, may be considered for splenectomy. Splenectomy usually restores the granulocyte levels to normal, temporarily, with gradual reappearance of neutropenia. Within several months to years after the operation, indolent infections usually recur. Chrysotherapy may be employed in some patients with care taken to monitor the leukocyte counts. Cytotoxic agents are contraindicated.

The disease should be distinguished from pyoderma gangrenosum and, most importantly, from SLE with rheumatoidlike features.

REFERENCES

1. Felty AR. Chronic arthritis in the adult, associated with splenomegaly and leukopenia: a report of five cases of an unusual clinical syndrome. Bull Johns Hopkins Hosp 35:16–20, 1924.
2. Ruderman M, Miller LM, Pinals RS. Clinical and serologic observations on 27 patients with Felty's syndrome. Arthritis Rheum 11:377–384, 1968.
3. Hurd ER, LaSpalluto J, Zill M. The role of immune complexes in production of the neutropenia of Felty's syndrome. J Rheumatol (Suppl 1) 1:105, 1974.

SJÖGREN'S SYNDROME

HARVEY E. BROWN, M.D.

Sjögren's syndrome is a chronic inflammatory process with diminished or absent secretion of lacrimal and salivary glands (1,2). It may be associated with classic rheumatoid arthritis (50% of cases) or some other connective tissue disease in the autoimmune category or in patients without any associated phenomena. Dryness of the mouth, xerostomia, and dry eyes, keratoconjunctivitis sicca, are associated with lymphocytic and plasma cell infiltration of glandular tissue (the sicca complex). In some, exocrine glands in the respiratory tract, gastrointestinal tract, or vagina may be involved. Lymphoid infiltrates may invade the lung or kidney.

The majority of patients are female, 50 years or older. The syndrome appears in all races. The sicca complex may appear in a patient with rheumatoid arthritis who has had arthritis for a considerable period of time or the development may be rapid with severe oral and ocular dryness in an otherwise normal person. Eye symptoms may begin with a gritty or sandy sensation. Thick, ropy strands of mucus at the inner canthus of the eye upon awakening may be distressing. Other symptoms include blepharitis and itching, photosensitivity, foggy vision, corneal ulceration, opacification, even perforation.

The persistent dry mouth may cause difficulty in chewing and swallowing or in phonation. Food adheres to the buccal surfaces. Fissures and ulcers of the tongue, mucus membranes, and lips appear, requiring frequent swallowing of liquids. Dental fillings may loosen and severe caries develop. The nasal mucosa may be dry, as well as the posterior pharynx, the larynx, and the tracheobronchial tree. Epistaxis, recurrent otitis media, bronchitis, or pneumonia may follow. A number of patients will have parotid gland enlargement. This may be recurrent and symmetric. It may be accompanied by fever, tenderness, or erythema.

Neuromuscular abnormalities include polymyositis and myopathy, peripheral or cranial neuropathy, and CNS vasculitis. Malignant lymphoproliferation or pseudolymphoma may be a late complication. Splenomegaly and vasculitis with leg ulcers may suggest Felty's syndrome. Raynaud's phenomenon has been reported in a few patients. A smaller number have chronic thyroiditis of the Hashimoto type.

The Schirmer filter paper test (Whatman #41) provides a practical measure of tear formation. More reliable diagnostic tests are associated with application of rose bengal dye and biomicroscopy. Small, superficial ulcers may be seen upon staining of the cornea. The erythrocyte sedimentation rate is elevated together with anemia, leukopenia, and hypergammaglobulinemia. Cryoglobulinemia may be present. A majority of patients have a positive rheumatoid factor, a slightly smaller percentage have antinuclear antibodies (homogeneous or speckled pattern), and yet a smaller number have LE cells in the blood.

The volume of parotid salivary flow may be measured directly, by secretory sialography with radiopaque contrast media, or by uptake, concentration and excretion of the radionuclide ^{99m}Tc-pertechnetate. Punch biopsy of the minor salivary glands may show significant lymphoid infiltration.

Treatment is symptomatic. Artificial tears may be helpful, as well as frequent ingestion of fluids. Meticulous oral hygiene is imperative. A moist and humid environment at home is supportive. The management of associated rheumatoid arthritis is similar to that of uncomplicated RA. Longevity usually is not affected. Corticosteroids or immunosuppressive drugs may be indicated with severe functional disability and for life-threatening complications. Malignant lymphoma should be treated with intensive chemotherapy.

REFERENCES

1. Shearn MA. Sjögren's Syndrome. Philadelphia: Saunders, 1971.
2. Mason AMS, Grumpel JN, Golding PL. Sjögren's syndrome: A clinical review. Semin Arthritis Rheum 4:301–331, 1973.
3. Dijkstra PF. Classification and differential diagnosis of sialographic characteristics in Sjögren syndrome. Semin Arthritis Rheum 10:10–17, 1973.

REITER'S SYNDROME

NORMAN L. GOTTLIEB, M.D.

Reiter's syndrome (RS), first described in 1916, is thought to be caused by an unidentified agent(s) that infects the genitourinary or gastrointestinal tract. The triad of nongonococcal urethritis, arthritis, and conjunctivitis are the characteristic manifestations of this syndrome. In addition, the skin, mucous, membranes, and nails may be affected. Most cases are sporadic, although epidemics have been reported, usually in association with bacillary dysentery.

Reiter's syndrome usually presents as acute arthritis and urethral discharge in 20- to 40-year-old men. This disorder is uncommonly diagnosed in women living in the United States, although recent evidence suggests it may occur more frequently than recognized (2). Associated systemic findings include fever, weight loss, diarrhea, anorexia, weakness, and fatigability (1).

CLINICAL FEATURES

The urethral discharge may be mucoid or mucopurulent, asymptomatic or associated with dysuria. Cultures for gonococci usually are negative, and gonococcal and Bedsonia antibodies are present in approximately the same frequency as in the venereal disease clinic population. Prostatitis, with a large, soft, tender gland from which many pus cells may be expressed, and hemorrhagic cystitis, usually associated with frequency, suprapubic pain, hematuria, and pyuria, may develop.

Articular involvement of RS is variable, but generally is asymmetric, polyarticular, and involves both large and small joints. Weight-bearing joints are affected more often than upper extremity joints.

Disease severity and duration and response to treatment vary greatly from patient to patient. One characteristic feature of RS that may be helpful diagnostically is the sausage digit, although diffusely swollen fingers and toes also may be seen with other rheumatoid variants such as psoriatic arthritis. Histologic examination of the synovial membrane shows edema, inflammatory cell infiltration. and proliferation of synovial lining cells, none of which permit differentiation from other inflammatory rheumatic conditions. The axial skeleton may be affected, showing only unilateral or bilateral sacroiliitis, or the findings of ankylosing spondylitis, as seen in Marie-Strümpell disease (Fig. 1). When the apophyseal joints of the axial skeleton are involved, back pain, stiffness, and limitation of motion may develop. Heel pain is common, resulting from Achilles tendinitis, plantar fasciitis, or bursitis.

Ocular involvement is common but frequently overlooked because symptoms are mild or transient. Conjunctivitis may be associated with

FIGURE 1

Sacroiliitis and asymmetric syndesmophyte formation are typical features of axial skeleton involvement in Reiter's syndrome.

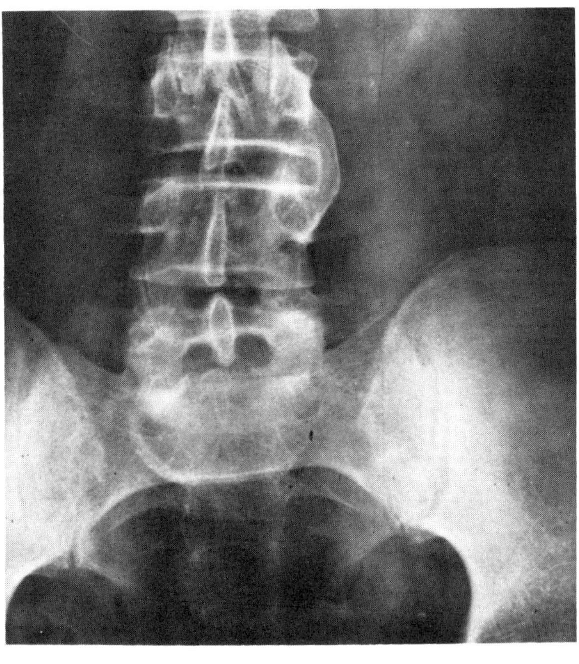

a mild burning sensation and a nonpurulent discharge. Iritis develops in 5 to 10% of patients during the initial attack and is seen more frequently in chronic RS. Keratitis, optic neuritis, retinitis, and macular edema are uncommon.

The skin often is involved in RS, dermatitis occurring most frequently on the palms of the hands and soles of the feet (Fig. 2). Keratoderma blennorrhagica usually develops several weeks after the onset of articular symptoms and generally is of short duration. The initial lesions are papular or pustular, discrete or confluent. When many lesions coalesce, a large area of skin may be covered with a thick keratotic crust that eventually peels without scar formation. Onycholysis and hyperkeratosis of the finger- and toenails may occur.

The most common mucous membrane lesions are superficial ulcer-

FIGURE 2
Keratoderma blennorrhagica on the soles of the feet in a patient with Reiter's syndrome.

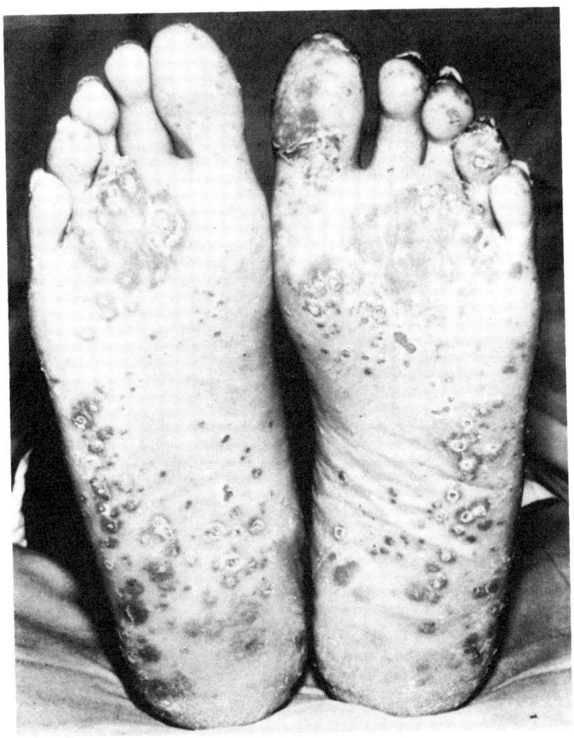

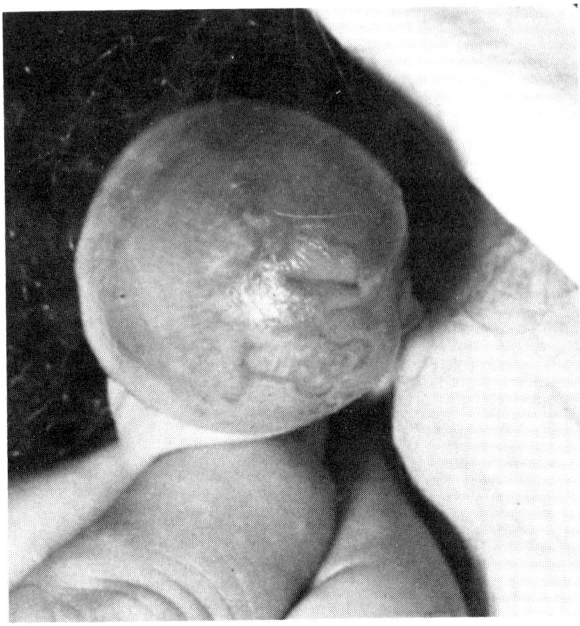

FIGURE 3
Balanitis circinata of the glans penis is one of several lesions affecting the genitals in Reiter's syndrome.

ations around the urethral meatus, balanitis circinata of the glans penis, and erythematous or ulcerative lesions of the buccal mucosa of the mouth and tongue (Fig. 3). The penile ulcerations may coalesce causing a circular or scalloped border, appear serpiginous, or mimic leutic disease. The oral mucosal lesions generally are small, superficial, painless, and asymptomatic; geographic tongue also has been noted.

Unusual, but serious complications of RS are pancarditis and valvular heart disease. Aortic insufficiency occurs in association with recurrent or prolonged arthritis and with electrocardiographic conduction defects, especially first degree atrioventricular block (3).

LABORATORY FINDINGS

Laboratory findings are not specific. Leukocytosis and anemia may develop in patients with chronic disease. Usually the erythrocyte sedimentation rate is elevated, at times markedly. The synovial fluid is turbid, cloudy, with an elevated white blood cell count (usually > $10,000/mm^3$) consisting largely of polymorphonuclear leukocytes, a normal glucose content, and a negative gram stain and culture for bacteria. Synovial fluid complement level may be elevated, and large macrophages with ingested WBC or RBC may be seen (4).

The histocompatibility antigen B27 is present in 75 to 95% of patients with RS, in contrast to 6 to 8% of the general population and patients with nonspecific urethritis and gonococcal arthritis (5, 6). Most RS patients with axial skeleton involvement and the traditional triad are B27 positive, whereas 66% of those with only peripheral arthritis and urethritis are HLA-B27 positive. HLA-B27 positive and B27 negative patients have similar clinical courses and response to treatment. Thus HLA-B27 may be a genetic marker for RS or part of some as yet undetermined mechanism associated with its etiology. Other seronegative spondyloarthropathies, such as ankylosing spondylitis, psoriatic arthritis, and yersinia arthritis, also are associated with a greater than anticipated frequency of HLA-B27, so that this relationship is not disease-specific.

COURSE AND TREATMENT

The course of RS is unpredictable; it may be acute, chronic, or intermittent. The majority of patients recover completely from the initial episode within several months, but others have prolonged illnesses with significant morbidity (7). Most patients have one or two additional attacks of RS within 2 years of the initial episode. Recent evidence indicates that 30% of patients develop long-term disability or permanent sequelae, suggesting that this disorder is not as benign as once considered (8). A small number of patients develop a syndrome indistinguishable from ankylosing spondylitis or psoriatic arthritis, whereas at the other end of the clinical spectrum, some have incomplete disease expression (9).

Although there is no specific treatment for RS, analgesics and antiinflammatory agents generally provide adequate symptomatic relief. Salicylates, indomethacin, phenylbutazone, and other newly marketed nonsteroidal antiinflammatory drugs have been used successfully. Patients unresponsive to these measures may benefit from intraarticular or systemic corticosteroids. Antibiotics generally are not helpful. Cytotoxic agents may prove beneficial in severely progressive cases, especially if vital organ systems are involved.

REFERENCES

1. Sharp JT. Reiter's syndrome. In: McCarty DJ, ed. Arthritis and Allied Conditions. Philadelphia: Lea & Febiger, 1979, 9th ed., p. 633.
2. Smith DL, Bennett RM, Regan MG. Reiter's disease in women. Arthritis Rheum 23:335-340, 1980.
3. Good AE. Reiter's disease. A review with special attention to cardiovascular and neurologic sequelae. Semin Arthritis Rheum 3:253-286, 1974.
4. Hasselbacher P. Immunoelectrophoretic assay for synovial fluid C3 with correction for synovial fluid globulin. Arthritis Rheum 22:243-250, 1979.
5. Brewerton DA, James DC. The histocompatibility antigen (HL-A27) and disease. Semin Arthritis Rheum 4:191-207, 1975.
6. Woodrow JC. Histocompatibility antigens and rheumatic diseases. Semin Arthritis Rheum 6:257-276, 1977.
7. Calin A. Reiter's syndrome. Med Clin North Am 61:365-376, 1977.
8. Fox R, Calin A, Gerber RC, et al. The chronicity of symptoms and disability in Reiter's syndrome. Ann Intern Med 91:190-193, 1979.
9. Arnett FC, McClusky OE, Schacter BZ, et al. Incomplete Reiter's disease: discriminating features and HLA-W27 in diagnosis. Ann Intern Med 84:8-12, 1976.

VIRAL ARTHRITIS

FRED H. HYER, M.D., AND NORMAN L. GOTTLIEB, M.D.

Viral arthritis usually develops as an acute self-limited, nondestructive process associated with other features of viral infection. Hepatitis B and rubella viruses are the most common recognized causes of viral arthritis in the United States; but many other viral agents produce articular inflammation (1,2).

Viral invasion and proliferation in synovial tissues is the apparent pathogenetic mechanism of mono- or pauciarticular viral arthritis. Viruses have been isolated from synovial fluid in patients with cytomegalovirus, rubella, herpes simplex, vaccinia, and varicella arthritis. In contrast, acute, symmetric polyarticular disease associated with hepatitis B and other viruses likely results from immune complex deposition in synovial and neighboring connective tissues. Lyme arthritis, a newly identified illness due to a putative arthropod-borne virus, is discussed in the next chapter.

HEPATITIS

The arthritis of viral hepatitis (1–3) is being diagnosed with increasing frequency due to greater physician awareness, the availability of laboratory tests for detecting hepatitis B antigens and antibodies, the higher prevalence of parenterally transmitted hepatitis (from drug abuse), and possibly the emergence of more "arthritogenic" strains of virus. The frequency of articular involvement in several reported series varies from 1.6% in children to 49% in adults. A realistic approximation is that 5 to 10% of hepatitis cases will manifest joint complaints. Females are affected more often than males in a ratio of 1.5:1.

The clinical presentation mimics acute serum sickness, with a transient, symmetric, sometimes migratory polyarthritis usually affecting the small joints of the hands, knees, and ankles. Approximately 50% of the cases are associated with pruritic dermatitis and low-grade fever. The rash and arthritis occur in the prodromal phase of hepatitis, preceding the clinical diagnosis of hepatitis by as long as 6 weeks.

Immunologic studies have shown markedly and consistently depressed total serum hemolytic complement and C4 levels, with a slightly reduced or normal C3 level. Synovial fluid complement levels similarly are depressed acutely. Electron microscopic studies have shown virallike particles in synovial lining and subsynovial cells and in synovial vessels. Thus an immunologic mechanism has been proposed for hepatitis arthritis, including circulating immune complexes (hepatitis B antigen-hepatitis B antibody), complement activation, and subsequent tissue inflammation.

RUBELLA

The synovitis that occurs after natural wild rubella virus infection most commonly is symmetric and polyarticular. It affects adolescents and adults primarily, follows the rash, and subsides in 1–2 weeks (2).

Vaccination with live attenuated rubella virus also may cause acute polyarthritis and is more common in the postpubertal population (3). Monoarticular disease, however, is seen in about 50% of cases. In one study of vaccinated adult women 43% developed arthralgias or arthritis 10–14 days later, symptoms lasting from 1 to 3 weeks. Rubella virus has been isolated from synovial fluid after natural infection and postvaccination. Synovianalysis shows a moderately inflammatory fluid (about 15,000 white blood cells/mm^3) with a predominance of mononuclear cells. Repeated bouts of arthritis followed rubella vaccination in one report of three children and was associated with persistent viral replication in the affected joints.

VARICELLA-ZOSTER

Varicella virus has been reported to cause a monoarthritis, pauciarthritis, or polyarthritis in children (1). The arthritis develops within 1 week of the appearance of the skin eruption and resolves spontaneously several days later. In one 8-year-old patient, varicella virus was cultured from knee fluid. Synovianalysis shows mildly inflammatory fluid with mononuclear cell predominance.

One case of herpes zoster was complicated by acute arthritis of both knees, which were warm, swollen, and tender (4). The synovial fluid white cell counts were 9000 and 2200/mm^3, the majority of which were polymorphonuclear leukocytes. Varicella virus was not detected by culture or electron microscopy, but varicella antigen was demonstrated in the cytoplasm of macrophages in the synovial fluid.

MUMPS

The prevalence of arthritis with mumps infection reportedly is less than 0.5%. The peak frequency occurs in the third decade of life; males predominate. Large joints are affected by an inflammatory process that usually begins the second week after onset of parotitis. Patients with mumps arthritis have a higher frequency of other extrasalivary manifestations such as orchitis, prostatitis, pancreatitis, and pericarditis. Salicylates generally provide unsatisfactory relief of arthritis symptoms, whereas ACTH is highly effective but does not shorten the disease course.

MYCOPLASMA

Mycoplasma pneumoniae has been reported in Great Britain to cause a rheumatoid fever-like illness. The diagnosis was established by rising cold agglutinin titers and complement fixation tests to *Mycoplasma pneumoniae.* A case of purulent monoarthritis of the knee was associated with a fourfold rise in antibody titers to *M. pneumoniae.*

SMALLPOX

Infection of bone and joint with smallpox virus develops in 2 to 5% of children and rarely in adults. A striking predilection for elbow involvement exists, occurring in 100% of one series of 15 Nigerian children. Severe arthritis, with joint crepitus, effusions, and draining sinuses is seen frequently; sometimes arthritis is associated with variola osteomyelitis. Variola arthritis is an exception to the rule that viral arthritis is benign.

ARTHRITIS ASSOCIATED WITH RESPIRATORY SYNDROMES

Eleven patients with acute upper respiratory symptoms, virallike in nature, developed synovitis in one series. All symptoms resolved spontaneously within 4 weeks. The knees were most commonly involved, followed by the metacarpophalangeal, proximal interphalangeal, and wrist joints. Synovial fluid analysis showed white blood cell counts ranging from 2800 to 24,800/mm^3, usually with a polymorphonuclear predominance. Rising serum antibody titers against numerous viruses could not be demonstrated in most patients.

MISCELLANEOUS

Polyarthritis has been associated with echo virus type 9 infection and EB virus in infectious mononucleosis (5). Monoarticular arthritis has been described recently in two patients with disseminated herpes simplex infection (6). In one, herpes simplex virus was isolated from knee joint fluid. Acute cytomegalovirus (CMV) monoarticular arthritis with virus recovery from knee fluid was reported in a postrenal transplant patient with generalized CMV infection (6).

Arthritis also has been reported with erythema infectiosum, a presumed viral disease. Sixty percent of adults developed articular symptoms in one epidemic in the state of Washington.

Acute tropical polyarthritis in certain African populations, Navajo arthritis, and New Guinea arthritis are of suspected viral etiology.

Mosquito-borne arbovirus infections causing inflammatory arthritis include Chikungunya and O'nyong-nyong in Africa and Ross River virus in Australia.

REFERENCES

1. Sauter SVH, Utsinger PD. Viral arthritis. Clin Rheum Dis 4:225–240, 1978.
2. Hyer FH, Gottlieb NL. Rheumatic disorders associated with viral infection. Semin Arthritis Rheum 8:17–31, 1978.
3. Steere AC, Malawista SE. Viral arthritis. In: McCarty DJ, ed. Arthritis and Allied Conditions. Philadelphia: Lea & Febiger, 1979, 9th ed., p. 139.
4. Cunningham AL, Fraser JRE, Clarris BJ, et al. A study of synovial fluid and cytology in arthritis associated with herpes zoster. Aust NZ J Med 9:440–443, 1979.

5. Blotzer JW, Myers AR. Echovirus-associated polyarthritis. Arthritis Rheum 21:978-981, 1978.
6. Friedman HM, Pincus T, Gibilisco P, et al. Acute monoarticular arthritis caused by herpes simplex virus and cytomegalovirus. Am J Med 69:241-247, 1980.

LYME DISEASE

HAL B. UNSCHULD, M.D., AND
NORMAN L. GOTTLIEB, M.D.

Lyme disease (LD), first described in 1976, is an epidemic, immune mediated inflammatory disorder that usually begins in the summer. A characteristic skin lesion, erythema chronicum migrans (ECM), is present in 85% of patients. Weeks to months later, rheumatologic (45%), neurologic (11%), or cardiac (8%) abnormalities may develop. This entity was recognized initially because of a tight geographic clustering of cases in eastern Connecticut. Subsequently, LD has been found in three distinct foci in the United States: the Northeast (Cape Cod, Massachusetts south to Maryland); the Midwest (Wisconsin); and the West (northern California and Oregon). The median age of onset is 16 years (range 2 to 71), with men and women affected with equal frequency. Substantial epidemiologic data suggest transmission of an unidentified (viral ?) agent by the tick vector, *Ixodes dammini* (1).

The following sequence of events has been postulated in the pathogenesis of LD. The etiologic factor is introduced into the skin by *I. dammini.* Three days to 3 weeks later, ECM develops at the tick bite site and circulating immune complexes are found. In genetically predisposed hosts, the immune response either fails to eradicate the agent or propagates itself by the continued elaboration of endogenous reactive material. In such patients, immune complexes disseminate, causing end-organ (e.g., articular, neurologic, cardiac) dysfunction (2).

CLINICAL MANIFESTATIONS

Erythema chronicum migrans is the best clinical marker for LD. The initial lesion, usually on a proximal extremity or on the trunk (most commonly the thigh, buttocks, or axilla), begins as a red macule or papule that expands to form a large annular lesion. Smaller secondary lesions develop in 50% of patients. The outer border of ECM typically is intensely red and flat; the middle often shows partial clearing; the center is sometimes indurated and a deeper red. The lesion usually is warm and fades within several weeks without residual pigmentary change. Frequently a burning sensation is present, but rarely pain or pruritus. No mucosal involvement has been described. Malaise, fatigue, fever, chills, headache, and stiff neck suggesting aseptic meningitis are common, while backache, myalgias, nausea, vomiting, and sore throat are less frequent. Lymphadenopathy, splenomegaly, erythematous tonsils, and other rashes may be found (3).

The arthritis of LD develops 4 days to 2 years (median 4 weeks) after the onset of ECM, although the skin lesion is sometimes absent. Synovitis usually begins suddenly in one or several joints and usually remains mono- or oligoarticular. In 25% of patients, migratory arthralgias may involve as many as 10 joints, followed by other large joints (shoulder, elbow), the TM joints, and occasionally small joints of the fingers and toes. Inflammation of a given joint characteristically is brief (median, 1 week), but many patients have recurrent attacks separated by longer periods of remission. Chronic arthritis occasionally develops in the knees, with pannus formation and cartilage and bone erosion. Typically the knees are swollen and warm, but seldom red. Ruptured popliteal (Baker's) cysts occur with some frequency, simulating thrombophlebitis. Swelling of other joints is less common, pain on motion often being the only sign of inflammation. Recurrence of prodromal symptoms is associated with recurrent arthritis attacks in 50% of patients. Joint fluid analysis shows elevation of the white blood cell count (median, 24,250/mm^3; range 2100 to 102,000), usually PMNs, and total protein of 3 to 8 gm (3).

Nervous system involvement occurs in 11% of patients, initial manifestations often developing while ECM is present and preceding arthritis. Neurologic syndromes include (1) aseptic meningitis with cerebrospinal fluid lymphocytic pleocytosis; (2) encephalitis and/or chorea; (3) cranial neuritis; (4) radiculoneuritis; and (5) myelitis. The usual pattern is multiple episodes of fluctuating meningoencephalitis with superimposed cranial and peripheral neuropathy or radiculopathy. The outcome is generally favorable, but 40% of patients have residual disabilities (4).

Approximately 8% of LD patients have cardiac involvement, which usually affects young adult males, occurs within 3 weeks of the onset of ECM, and is of brief duration (3 days to 6 weeks). The most common abnormality is varying degrees of AV block manifest as fluctuating 1° block, Wenckebach type 2 block, and complete heart block. Other patients demonstrate EKG changes consistent with myopericarditis. Valvular heart disease is not a consequence of LD (5).

LABORATORY DATA

The red and white blood cell counts are usually normal, but hematocrits as low as 33% and WBC counts up to $16{,}000/mm^3$ with a marked left shift have been observed. As many as 10% atypical lymphocytes have been found. The following tests are normal or negative: urinalysis, BUN, creatinine, liver function tests, Australia antigen, infectious mononucleosis monospot, FANA, and rheumatoid fever. The erythrocyte sedimentation rate usually is elevated during attacks. Cultures of body fluids have been negative, and serological data have failed to implicate any known organism as the etiologic agent.

Two immunologic markers for LD have been identified. First, the B-cell alloantigen DRw-2 occurs in 70% of patients with chronic LD, whereas it is present in 22% of the general population. Second, the presence of IgM cryoprecipitates (immune complexes) in the serum during active ECM strongly correlates with the subsequent development of neurologic, rheumatologic, or cardiac disease. The presence of cryoglobulins, increased IgM concentrations, and decreased IgG concentrations correlate well with disease activity. C_3 and C_4 levels remain normal or increase slightly during active disease. With chronic arthritis, immune complexes are uniformly found in joint fluid but uncommonly in serum.

TREATMENT

Antibiotic (particularly penicillin G or tetracycline, but not erythromycin) treatment with active ECM for 7–10 days causes more rapid resolution of ECM and its associated symptoms. Although the frequency of subsequent neurologic and cardiac problems is not affected by antibiotics, fewer penicillin-treated patients develop arthritis and the duration of arthritis is shorter. Salicylates, nonsteroidal antiinflammatory agents, systemic and intraarticular corticosteroids, and synovectomy have been used to alleviate joint symptoms, with variable results (6). Meningeal signs usually are suppressed rapidly by oral prednisone (40-60 mg/day); encephalitic signs respond less well. After laboratory tests have returned to normal, residual neurologic deficits did not benefit from continued steroid therapy (4).

Patients with high degree AV block or 1° block with a PR interval of greater than 0.30 sec should be hospitalized because of the marked risk of complete heart block. A temporary cardiac pacemaker, aspirin, and prednisone have been used to treat complete-heart block. Patients with slight prolongation of the PR interval may be followed as outpatients while on restricted activity (5).

REFERENCES

1. Steere, AC, Malawista SE. Cases of Lyme disease in the United States: locations correlated with distribution of Ixodes dammini. Ann Intern Med 91:730-733, 1979.
2. Hardin AJ, Steere AC, Malawista SE. Immune complexes and the evolution of Lyme arthritis: dissemination and localization of abnormal c1q binding activity. N Engl J Med 301:1358-1363, 1979.
3. Steere AC, Malawista SE, Hardin JA, Ruddy S, Askenase PW, Andiman WA. Erythema chronicum migrans and Lyme arthritis: the enlarging clinical spectrum. Ann Intern Med 86:685-698, 1977.
4. Reik L, Steere AC, Bartenhagen NH, Shope RE, Malawista SE. Neurologic abnormalities of Lyme disease. Medicine 58:281-294, 1979.
5. Steere AC, Batsford WP, Weinberg M, et al. Lyme carditis: cardiac abnormalities of Lyme disease. Ann Intern Med 93:8-16, 1980.
6. Steere AC, Malawista SE, Newman JH, Spieler PN, Bartenhagen NH. Antibiotic therapy in Lyme disease. Ann Intern Med 93:1-8, 1980.

SYSTEMIC LUPUS ERYTHEMATOSUS

ROY D. ALTMAN, M.D.

Systemic lupus erythematosus (SLE) is a chronic multisystem disease characterized by episodes of clinical activity interspersed with episodes of complete or near complete remission. The notion that lupus is an acute, rapidly fatal illness in all instances is no longer tenable. Instances of a relatively benign form with limited involvement of a few organs are now recognized. In addition, earlier recognition and the use of corticosteroids have improved the prognosis greatly. In a prospective study by Estes and Christian (1), 50% of the patients were alive after 10 years. SLE is a disease of adolescents and young adults with a strong predilection for females (80–90% of patients). Overemphasis of this fact has resulted in needless delay in the diagnosis in middle-aged males and females afflicted with the disorder. The etiology of lupus remains unresolved.

Discoid lupus erythematosus (DLE) is a chronic disease of the skin. It appears by current concepts to comprise the same disease as SLE and represents the most benign end of the spectrum of clinical presentations. Numerous permutations between the all-cutaneous and systemic forms of the disease have been reported. The incidence of conversion from uncomplicated DLE to a more systemic form is less than 10%.

CLINICAL DIAGNOSIS

The American Rheumatism Association in 1971 published preliminary criteria for classification of SLE. The following criteria were proposed for the purpose of classifying patients in clinical trials, population surveys, and similar studies. A patient was considered to have SLE if any four or more of the following 14 manifestations are present, serially or simultaneously, during any interval of observation.

1. FACIAL ERYTHEMA (BUTTERFLY RASH). Diffuse erythema, flat or raised, over the malar eminence(s) and/or bridge of the nose; may be unilateral (Fig. 1).
2. DISCOID LUPUS. Erythematous raised patches with adherent keratotic sealing and follicular plugging; atrophic scarring may occur in older lesions; may be present anywhere on the body.
3. RAYNAUD'S PHENOMENON. Requires a two-phase color reaction: patient's history or physician's observation.

FIGURE 1

SLE facial rash. Note facial blush with butterfly distribution of raised, infiltrated, and hyperpigmented lesions with sparing of the nasolabial folds.

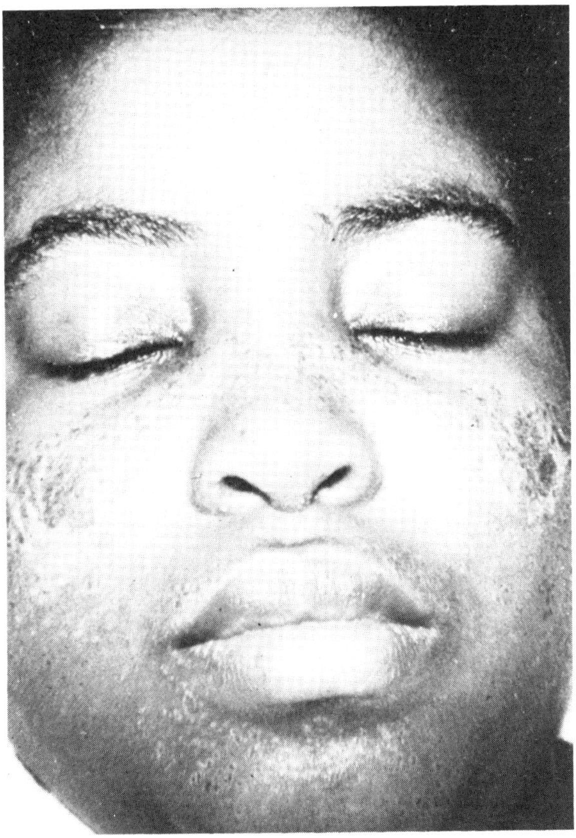

4. ALOPECIA. Rapid loss of large amount of scalp hair: patient's history or physician's observation (Fig. 2).
5. PHOTOSENSITIVITY. Unusual skin reaction from exposure to sunlight: patient's history or physician's observation.
6. ORAL OR NASOPHARYNGEAL ULCERATION.
7. ARTHRITIS WITHOUT DEFORMITY. One or more peripheral joints involved with any of the following in the absence of deformity.
    a. Pain on motion
    b. Tenderness
    c. Effusion or periarticular soft tissue swelling (peripheral joints are defined for this purpose as feet, ankles, knees, hips,

FIGURE 2

SLE scalp. Note forehead alopecia in this young female. The short, stubby hairs are characteristic of a lupus forelock.

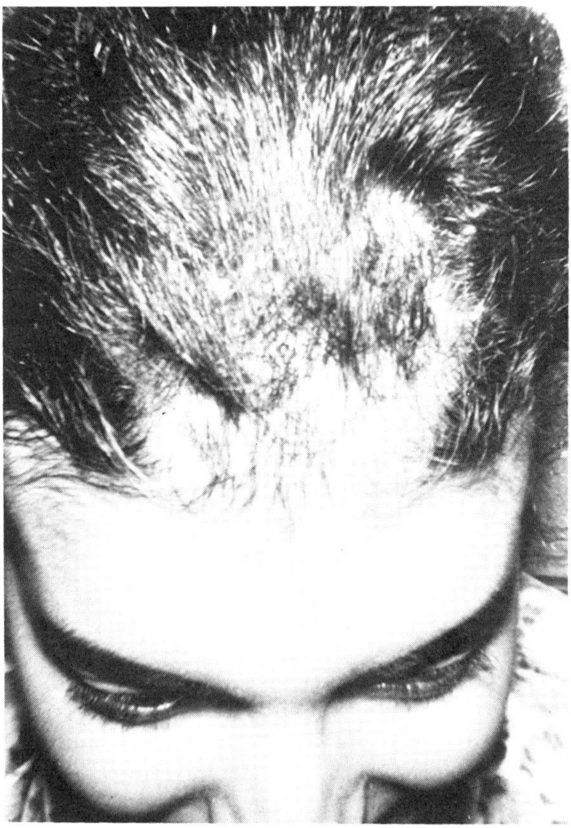

shoulders, elbows, wrists, metacarpophalangeal, proximal interphalangeal, terminal interphalangeal, and temporomandibular joints).

8. LE CELLS. Two or more classic LE cells seen on one occasion or one cell seen on two or more occasions, using an accepted published method.
9. CHRONIC FALSE-POSITIVE STS. Known to be present for at least 6 months and confirmed by TPI or Reiter's tests.
10. PROFUSE PROTEINURIA. Greater than 3.5 mg/day.
11. CELLULAR CASTS. May be red cell, hemoglobin, granular, tubular, or mixed.
12. ONE OR BOTH OF THE FOLLOWING:
    a. Pleuritis, with a history of pleuritic pain; or rub heard by physician; or x-ray evidence of both pleural thickening and fluid.
    b. Pericarditis, documented by EKG or rub.
13. ONE OR BOTH OF THE FOLLOWING:
    a. Psychosis
    b. Convulsions, by patient's history or physician's observation, in the absence of uremia and offending drugs.
14. ONE OR MORE OF THE FOLLOWING:
    a. Hemolytic anemia
    b. Leukopenia, WBC less than $4000/mm^3$ on two or more occasions.
    c. Thrombocytopenia, platelet count less than $100{,}000/mm^3$.

CLINICAL SYNDROME

The joint and periarticular manifestations of SLE are most often arthralgias rather than true arthritis. When synovitis occurs, it most often leaves no residual deformity. SLE should be suspected if rheumatoid arthritis is diagnosed and the involved joints remain free of erosions for 2 or more years. The transitory nature of the polyarthralgia and arthritis early in SLE is important. A common complaint is morning stiffness with diffuse hand puffiness that subsides in minutes to hours. At this stage there may be a normal sedimentation rate, although LE cells and a significant titer of antinuclear antibodies are found (2). If joint fluid is obtained it usually has high viscosity and a good mucin clot. There may be low complement and LE cells in the fluid. Deformity can occur, although it is not associated with pannus or erosions and deformity is readily reducible. Muscle complaints and weakness are common, but a true proximal myopathy with weakness is seen in less than 5% of cases. When found, consideration should be given to a causal role of corticosteroid or antimalarial therapy.

Cardiac involvement may occur, especially with pericarditis, with or without pericardial effusion. Cardiac tamponade is uncommon; when it does develop it generally responds promptly to massive doses of glucocorticoids (1000 mg of hydrocortisone or its equivalent in 24 hr). Rarely, pericardiocentesis is required. A complication of therapy in SLE is development of premature arteriosclerotic heart disease, seemingly related to long-term and high dose glucocorticoid therapy. Similarly, hypertension is common, in some due to corticosteroid therapy and in others due to progressive renal involvement. Libman-Sacks endocarditis is rarely clinically significant.

The lung may be involved with pneumonitis, pleuritis with or without effusion, and, less commonly, fibrosis. The sugar concentration in pleural fluid tends to be normal in contrast to low glucose often seen in the pleural effusions of rheumatoid arthritis. Even without x-ray changes, there may be impaired pulmonary function with reduced diffusion capacity. A few patients develop chronic idiopathic pulmonary fibrosis. Lupus pneumonitis is uncommon but presents a difficult differential diagnosis with infection when it does occur. Early lung biopsy through bronchoscopy or open lung biopsy may help establish diagnosis.

The kidneys are involved in more than 50% of patients. Findings include mesangial glomerulonephritis, focal glomerulonephritis, diffuse glomerulonephritis, membranous glomerulonephritis, and fibrotic glomerulonephritis (3). Urine sediment is a poor predictor of histologic change. Renal biopsy may be needed for clarification of prognosis and planning therapy. Although proteinuria does not predict outcome, an active urine sediment (cells and casts) with azotemia does portend a poor prognosis irrespective of the biopsy findings. Mesangial changes alone carry the best prognosis. Diffuse proliferative changes with crescents as well as fibrotic glomeruli predict the poorest prognosis. In those with seemingly normal kidneys, renal biopsies are abnormal in 50%. With seemingly normal renal function, evidence of renal tubular acidosis may be detected, especially with an acid loading test. There appears to be a correlation between increasing urinary L chain output, decreasing complement levels, and active renal disease.

The nervous system is involved in at least 50% of patients, theoretically due to microinfarcts and small blood vessel disease (5). There may be focal signs or mental deterioration. The latter may be confused with glucocorticoid side effects. There may be peripheral neuropathy, seizures, psychosis, mononeuritis multiplex, or a variety of neurologic findings. There are no current consistent criteria to diagnose CNS lupus. The presence of cortical atrophy on computer assisted tomography of the skull in a young patient predicts serious cortical disease related directly to the SLE.

Ocular findings are present in 50% of patients, consisting usually of filamentary keratitis with a positive Schirmer's test greater than 5 but less than 10 mm. Sjögren's syndrome is common. Cytoid bodies are uncommon.

Hematologically, anemia and leukopenia are seen in 50% of the patients, severe thrombocytopenia in less than 10%. Leukopenia is often a guide to activity of disease. Thrombocytopenia is due to an antibody for platelets; the anemia, if severe and not related to renal failure, is commonly associated with an antibody for red cells and is Coombs' positive. Occasionally, autoimmune hemolytic anemia and thrombocytopenia coexist or occur alternately in the same patient. This syndrome (Evan's syndrome) is usually due to SLE. Patients with SLE often have one or another hematologic abnormality. The most common and most nonspecific is anemia, which may be secondary to a chronic inflammatory process. Many patients have leukopenia, which may involve all forms of white blood cells, although total counts below 2000 MM^3 are unusual. A Coombs' positive hemolytic anemia is seen in 5 to 10% of patients and is usually responsive to corticosteroids. Splenectomy is of little value in controlling this complication. On occasion, thrombocytopenia may be a prominent feature (it may be the first manifestation). In any young individual who presents with thrombocytopenia, SLE, idiopathic thrombocytopenia, and drug-induced thrombocytopenia should be considered (6). A bleeding diathesis due to circulating anticoagulants occurs in some patients with SLE.

Involvement of the skin occurs in 80% of patients. Numerous types of skin involvement can occur, including those described in the classification of SLE. In addition, one may see vascular ulcers about the ankles or elbows, Henoch-Shöenlein appearing purpura, palmar vasculitis, eythema multiforme, toxic epidermal necrolysis, and others. Biopsy of involved as well as uninvolved skin may show immunoglobulin staining for complement and IgG. Biopsy of the vascular lesion often shows the characteristic leukocytoclastic angiitis. Mucous membrane lesions occur in 20%. Flare-ups of skin involvement are frequently associated with systemic exacerbations of the disease. Variable loss of hair is seen in 33% of patients. Hair loss is commonly associated with active disease. Most frequently one sees spotty alopecia areata or forehead hair loss with a forelock of short, stubby hair. Aseptic necrosis, especially in hips or knees, can occur in SLE with or without corticosteroid therapy, usually in young patients and within 4 years of diagnosis.

Several precipitating factors may be associated with the onset or exacerbation of the disease such as exposure to sunlight, infection, acute emotional stress, or drugs (e.g., tetanus antitoxin, gold, sulfonamides, and antibiotics such as penicillin).

The results of controlled family studies confirm a higher frequency of connective tissue disease and/or serologic abnormalities (ANA, RF) among relatives than among controls, but not necessarily an increased incidence of SLE.

There is considerable evidence implicating immunologic mechanisms in the pathogenesis. Studies have documented the deposition of immunoglobulins and complement in many organs and vessels (in choroid plexus, along basement membrane in both subepithelial and subendothelial locations in the kidney, in vessels of spleen, lungs, and heart, and in skin along basement membrane). In addition, there is good evidence implicating anti-DNA complexed with DNA in the pathogenesis of lupus glomerulonephritis. This action is mediated by the fixation of complement, which leads to chemotaxis, accumulation of neutrophils, phagocytosis of complexes, and subsequent rupture of these cells and release of toxic substances. In addition, thrombocytopenia and hemolytic anemia are secondary to autoimmune phenomena. Patients with active disease frequently demonstrate low serum and synovial fluid complement.

Protein abnormalities are common. Hypergammaglobulinemia is characteristic. Some patients demonstrate cryoglobulins, which may play a clinical role (Raynaud's phenomenon, purpura, abdominal crises). A positive RA latex occurs in as many as 40% of patients.

Considerable study has been devoted to the elaboration of antibodies in SLE, particularly the antinuclear antibodies (ANA). These are between 15 and 20 well-defined antibodies to nuclear components. It is only a matter of time before a sensitive and specific test for SLE will be available commercially. At present the antinuclear antigen is most commonly determined by an immunofluorescent technique that employs animal nuclei, the patient's serum, and human gammaglobulin tagged with fluorescence. Most patients with active SLE will have high titers of ANA, usually in a peripheral or rim pattern. Inactive SLE may be associated with a homogenous pattern. More than 90% of patients have detectable ANA. Subsets of SLE, e.g., C_{1q} deficiency, comprise a portion of the ANA negative patients. Antidouble stranded DNA antibodies seem most characteristic of SLE. These are most commonly determined by either nuclear (Farr technique) or immunofluorescent (Crithidia) techniques. Both methods are moderately sensitive and specific.

Many drugs can induce an SLE-like syndrome, most notably hydralazine, methyldopa, chlorpromazine, and, especially, procainamide. In procainamide-induced SLE, a positive ANA is always found and LE cells are present in most cases. Antideoxyribonucleoprotein is frequently present as is RF. Antinative DNA and antidenatured DNA are found in authentic SLE, but only the latter has been described rarely in procainamide-induced SLE. Also, in procainamide-induced SLE, complement is not depressed. The skin and kidneys are uncommonly involved.

PROGNOSIS

The prognosis in SLE is determined by renal, neurologic, and infectious complications. These three factors account for the majority of deaths. Renal involvement is the most common cause of death. If a patient is to develop renal disease, it will often occur within 5 years of the diagnosis of SLE. Histologically, nephritis is focal, membranous (wire-loop), or proliferative. Focal nephritis carries a good prognosis, membranous nephritis can be associated with little functional impairment, and proliferative nephritis usually carries a poor prognosis even with treatment. Hypertension is an indicator of serious renal involvement and usually appears when the patient becomes uremic.

Neurologic complications account for as many as 25% of deaths, usually as organic brain syndrome with secondary infection. In addition, death may occur from status epilepticus or intracerebral hemorrhage. The clinical features may include one or more of the following: mental disturbance (e.g., personality disorders, psychosis), grand mal seizures, hemiparesis, and cranial nerve signs. Peripheral neuropathies are uncommon. Convulsions may be accompanied by increased spinal fluid protein and pleocytosis. Infection is becoming an increasing cause of death since the introduction of corticosteroid therapy.

THERAPY

The treatment of SLE involves the judicious use of general measures that prevent complications. Sunscreens or avoidance of sunlight are recommended for patients with photosensitivity. Prophylactic medication such as antibiotics should be avoided because of the high incidence of hypersensitivity reactions. When in remission, patients may require no therapy.

Salicylates may be of value in controlling patients with mild disease such as predominantly joint symptoms. Antimalarials are valuable in the treatment of mild disease, especially in patients with skin lesions resulting from photosensitivity. These agents are less valuable in severely ill patients. In addition, antimalarials are associated with significant side effects. Listed in order of decreasing frequency, these are dermatitis, corneal opacities that are usually reversible, retinal damage that may not be reversible, and bone marrow depression.

Corticosteroids remain the mainstay of therapy for severely ill patients. These agents have improved survival and quality of life. However, they are associated with significant side effects and are not uniformly effective in the treatment of renal or neurologic manifestations.

Immunosuppressive agents are indicated when patients are not responding to corticosteroids or display serious side effects from them. They may have value in reducing requirements for corticosteroids. Their role in treatment of this disease is unclear. Several studies have questioned their value in lupus renal disease.

Cytotaxic agents that are most commonly used in severe SLE are cyclophosphamide (Cytoxan) and azathioprine (Imuran). Both agents have been used extensively but studied efficiently only in SLE renal disease. Cytoxan appears to be more effective as an immunosuppressive, whereas Imuran appears effective as an antiinflammatory agent. Vinblastine (Oncovin) has been used successfully for thromboajtopenia of various etiologies. On occasion, the patient's platelets can be incubated with Oncovin and returned to the patient as a potent killer of macrophages.

Recent clinical research has utilized intermittent bolus amounts of corticosteroids such as methylprenisolone acetate (Medrol) 1 g intravenously at intervals of 1 week to 1 month. Although preliminary data on plasmapheresis appears promising, it is presently an expensive research tool.

REFERENCES

1. Estes D, Christian CL. The natural history of systemic lupus erythematosus by prospective analysis. Medicine 50:85-95, 1971.
2. Dubois EL. Current status of the LE cell test. Semin Arthritis Rheum 1:97-115, 1971.
3. Baldwin DS, Lowenstein J, Rothfield NF, et al. The clinical course of the proliferative and membranous forms of lupus nephritis. Ann Intern Med 73:929-942, 1970.
4. Baldwin DS, Gluck MC, Lowenstein J, et al. Lupus nephritis clinical course as related to morphologic forms and their transitions. Am J Med 62:12-30, 1977.
5. Baker M. Psychopathology in systemic lupus erythematosus: I. Psychiatric observations. Semin Arthritis Rheum 3:95-110, 1973.
6. Fish AJ, Blau EB, Westberg NG, et al. Systemic lupus erythematosus within the first two decades of life. Am J Med 62:99-117, 1977.

ACUTE DERMATOMYOSITIS-POLYMYOSITIS

JOHN H. TALBOTT, M.D.

The terms acute dermatomyositis and polymyositis (AD-P) frequently are synonymous. Clinical findings are similar except for dermatitis in AD. This disease (or diseases) appears as a diffuse inflammatory disorder of striated skeletal muscle that causes symmetric weakness and atrophy principally of the central groups of muscles, shoulder girdle, pelvic girdle, neck, and pharynx, with involvement of one or more internal organs. It has been observed in infants as well as late in life. There may be considerable overlapping in well-developed cases with certain features of the other collagen-vascular diseases, sometimes with SLE, in others with progressive systemic sclerosis (PSS) or periarteritis nodosa (PN). In adults, but not in children, there is a significant incidence of an associated neoplasm without any preferred organ site. On the other hand, children may develop fatal vasculitis (1).

PATHOGENESIS

The cause of AD-P is not known (2). Infectious agents have been suspected but not proved. Viruslike structures have been seen in muscle cells or tubular inclusions resembling nucleocapsids of paramyxovirus in myocytes and endothelial cells of vessels in skin. The casual association with malignant tumors in some cases has led to the theory that the neoplasm induces the changes in the muscle through an immunologic or hypersensitivity reaction. In this context the myositis may be the result of an autoimmune reaction directed against the antigens common to the tumor and the muscle. The association of inflammatory myopathy with autoantibodies to nuclear antigens and clinical features of such diseases as SLE and Sjögren's syndrome lends support to this concept. Deposits of Ig, IgM, and C3 have been found in blood vessel walls, especially in children.

PATHOLOGY

The cardinal feature of polymyositis is inflammatory cellular infiltration with necrosis of muscle fibers as seen on muscle biopsy. The site for biopsy may be determined by electrical abnormalities. The quadriceps femoris or the deltoid usually show focal or extensive primary degeneration of fibers. Features of regeneration may be near areas of necrosis (Fig. 1). Focal or diffuse infiltrates of chronic inflammatory cells may be seen near blood vessels or between individual muscle fibers. As the disease progresses, interstitial fibrosis as well as variation in cross-sectional diameter of the fibers may appear.

FIGURE 1

Skeletal muscle from a biopsy specimen of a female who had symptoms of polymyositis for 6 months. Focal inflammatory changes and patchy fibrosis between involved muscle bundles are seen.

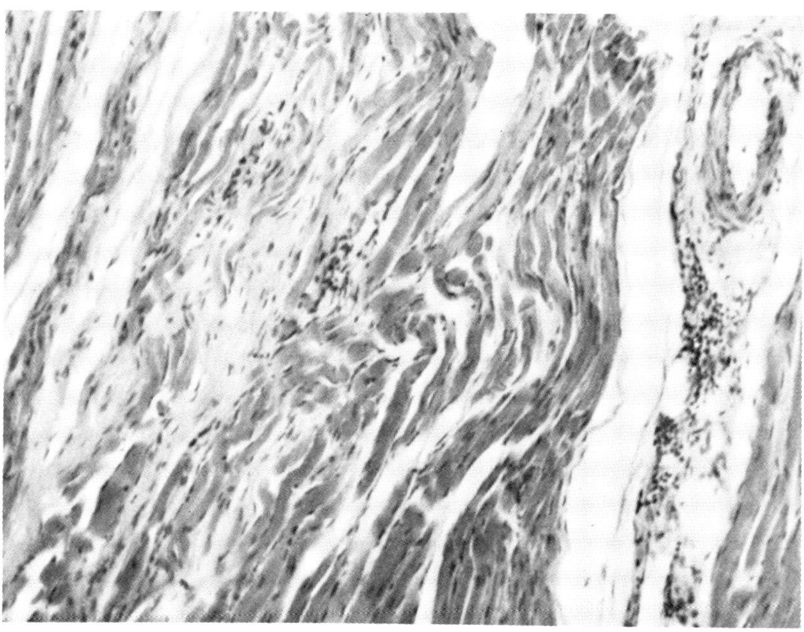

CLINICAL FEATURES

AD-P is not a rare disease. Incidence is greatest in females. The presenting symptoms may suggest RA or acute rheumatic fever with intermittent, low grade fever, malaise, and fatigability. In other cases, the profound muscle weakness that causes the patient to seek medical help is similar to that of severe myasthenia gravis, acute adrenal insufficiency, or pseudobulbar palsy. Weight loss may be rapid concomitant with swallowing difficulties and weakness in the pelvic and shoulder girdle. Proximal muscle weakness occurs in as many as 95% of patients, dysphasia in 50%, and weakness of the neck muscles in a smaller percentage. Distal muscle involvement may be as low as 20%. Skin lesions are present in a majority of patients; some may complain of Raynaud's phenomenon or arthralgias (Fig. 2).

The patient may have difficulty in standing up after sitting or getting out of a bathtub. A high bus step may be impossible to reach;

FIGURE 2

Hands of a patient who developed acute central muscle weakness 3.5 years after a carcinoma of the breast had been removed surgically. Ulnar deviation of the right and patchy synovitis of the PIP joints are seen.

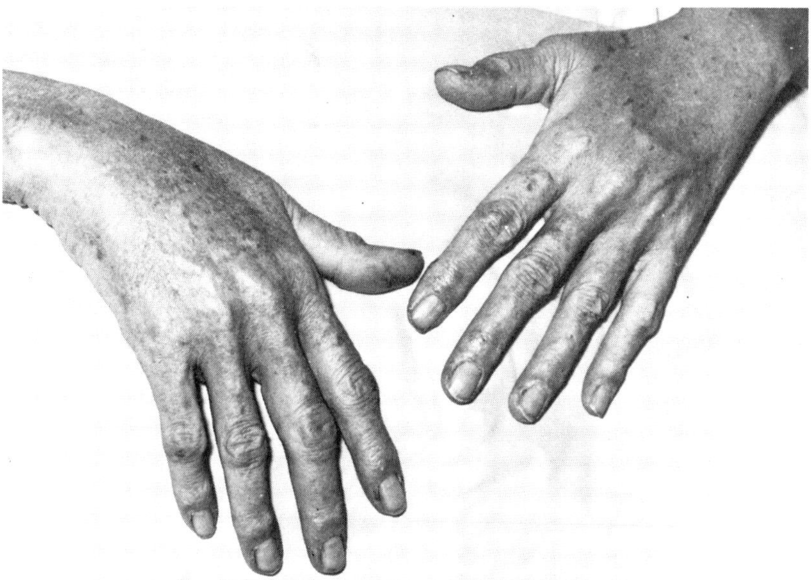

stairs may be ascended only by holding a handrail. The gait becomes clumsy from pelvic girdle weakness. At times the shoulder girdle is principally involved. Combing the hair with elevation of the arms is difficult or impossible. Involvement of the anterior neck muscle may be evident by the inability to raise the head from the pillow. Involvement of the posterior pharyngeal muscles may be responsible for dysphasia and dysphonia. Contractures or shortening of skeletal muscles are late manifestations, more common in children than in adults.

The characteristic skin rash is a dusky red or heliotrope color most evident about the eyes, with edema of the lids. It may also have a butterfly pattern of distribution (Fig. 3). The rash may also be seen on

FIGURE 3
Purplish brown pigmentation of the eyelids and telangiectasia in the patient whose hands are shown in Figure 2.

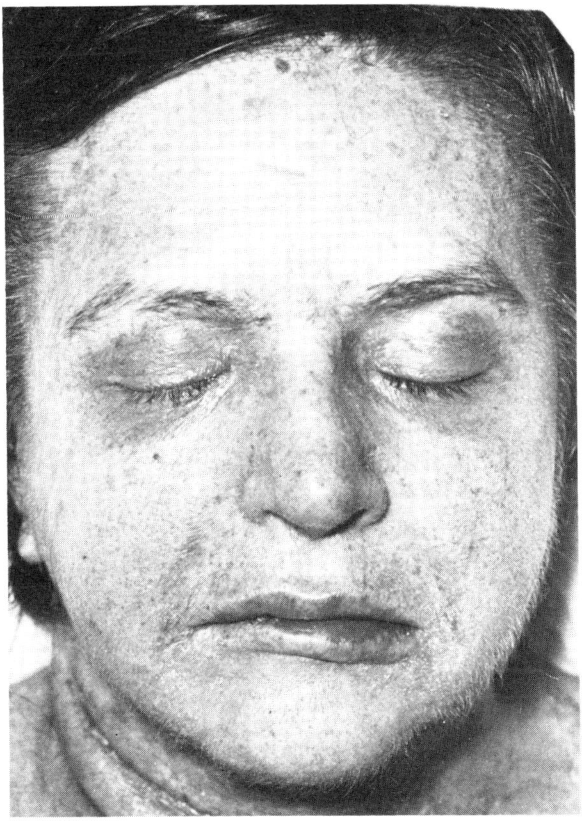

the V of the neck, on the elbows, over the dorsum of the interphalangeal or metacarpophalangeal joints, over the knees, and on the medial malleoli of the ankles. It is slightly elevated and sometimes scaly. There may be hyperemia of the fingertips.

Internal involvement may include the lungs, gastrointestinal tract, and heart. Several of the gastrointestinal tract changes may be similar to those of PSS; a smaller percentage develop pulmonary fibrosis. The weakness or paralysis of the posterior pharyngeal musculature is evident from difficulty or inability to swallow, sometimes even liquids. A barium swallow may be regurgitated into the trachea or slowly propelled into the esophagus where peristalsis is delayed. Atrophy of the muscularis of the large bowel, with formation of sacculations and huge diverticulae have been observed. There may be extensive subcutaneous calcinosis as in PSS. The development of this complication seems to be less common at present because of the widespread use of corticosteroids.

Children with AD may have abdominal pain, hematemesis, and melena, the result of widespread gastrointestinal vasculitis and ulcerations that may lead to perforation and death (1).

MALIGNANCY

The frequency of coexistent malignant disease in some series is as high as 20%, or from four to five times that expected on the basis of chance in an age-matched population. Coexistent tumors have not been observed in afflicted children. The time interval between discovery of a malignancy and clinical evidence of AD-P or between onset of symptoms of AD-P and later a malignancy, may be as long as 5 years. When a diagnosis of AD-P is made in an adult, especially over the age of 50, a careful search should be conducted for an accompanying malignancy. The malignancy may involve the lungs, prostate, ovaries, uterus, pancreas, intestines, etc. Removal or successful treatment of the malignancy may be associated with significant but usually only temporary improvement in various manifestations of the disease.

LABORATORY FINDINGS

Most of the usual laboratory tests are normal except for elevation of the ESR and muscle enzymes. A neutrophilic leukocytosis may occur; anemia is unusual. ANA or LE cells are not found. A low titer for RF may be present. Several of the muscle enzymes may be elevated significantly. These include the transaminases, creatine phosphokinase, dehydrogenase, and aldolase, indicators of muscle injury. This knowledge is useful in prognosis and in assessing the therapeutic effect of a drug or confirming an apparent spontaneous remission. Myoglobulinemia and myoglobulinuria of mild degree may be observed.

Electromyographic findings are helpful in establishing the diagnosis as well as the site for biopsy. A characteristic triad may be observed. This includes spontaneous fibrillation and positive saw-tooth potentials, complex polyphasic or short duration potentials on voluntary contraction, and salvos of repetitive high frequency action potentials (3).

PROGNOSIS

Prognosis is generally better in children than in adults. In one series, the overall cumulative survival after a 7-year follow-up period was 53% for adults and 90% for children. A malignancy may alter the prognosis critically.

TREATMENT

Treatment is relatively satisfactory. It consists of supportive therapy with corticosteroids and in some cases with immunosuppressive or cytotoxic agents. Adults should receive prednisone in divided doses as high as 80 to 150 mg/day, initially, until acute symptoms regress. Serial analyses of serum enzyme levels may be a guide to determining effectiveness of this therapy. If enzyme levels fall, encouragement is justified. The prednisone dosage is reduced slowly while monitoring the enzyme levels. Continued maintenance therapy with 10 to 20 mg of prednisone daily may be necessary. Methotrexate, 25 to 50 mg daily, has been used to supplement corticosteroids or to reduce the daily amount of prednisone formerly needed.

REFERENCES

1. Banker BQ, Victor M. Dermatomyositis (systemic angiopathy) of childhood. Medicine 45:261-289, 1966.
2. Talbott JR. Acute dermatomyositis-polymyositis with malignancy. Semin Arthritis Rheum 6:305-360, 1977.
3. Pearson CM, Bohan A. The spectrum of polymyositis and dermatomyositis. Med Clin North Am 61:439-457, 1977.

POLYARTERITIS

NORMAN L. GOTTLIEB, M.D.

The term polyarteritis nodosa (PAN) originally was used to describe a rare systemic illness in which palpable nodules of medium-size arteries, skin, and internal organs were found at postmortem examination. Since the nodular lesions frequently were absent, the term polyarteritis was adapted; others prefer "necrotizing angiitis" because the venous system may also be involved. Pathologically, polyarteritis is characterized by inflammation and fibrinoid necrosis of medium and small arteries (1).

ETIOLOGY

The etiology of PAN is unknown, although hypersensitivity is a favored hypothesis. Whereas adverse drug reactions, especially from sulfonamides and antibiotics, have been temporally related to the development of PAN, the majority of cases lack a history of drug sensitization. Immunologic studies suggest that vascular damage in PAN results from immune complex deposition. Polyarteritis has been associated with hepatitis B (HB) antigenemia or HB antibody in approximately 50% of cases and with acute serous otitis media (2,3). Immunofluorescent techniques have demonstrated immunoglobulins, complement and HB antigen in blood vessel walls, liver cell nuclei, kidney glomeruli, and other structures (4).

CLINICAL MANIFESTATIONS

Polyarteritis affects men 3 times more frequently than women; the peak age of onset is between 20 and 50 years of age. The clinical manifestations of PAN are protean in nature, depending upon the organ system(s) involved and the severity of involvement (5). It may begin abruptly or gradually, presenting as fever of unknown origin, hypertension, renal failure, peripheral neuropathy, or gastrointestinal disease. Renal involvement occurs in approximately 75% of cases, the most common findings including proteinuria and hematuria; hypertension is present in a smaller percentage. The relationship between renal histopathology, which frequently exhibits changes of arteritis and glomerulonephritis, and hypertension is unclear.

Abdominal pain, often severe, may be accompanied by other gastrointestinal symptoms such as nausea, diarrhea, and bloody stools and frequently is mistaken for more common bowel disorders. Mucosal ulceration with hemorrhage or perforation, mesenteric arteritis with thrombosis and infarction of bowel, or involvement of the gallbladder, pancreas, etc. are seen pathologically.

Pulmonary manifestations include hemorrhagic effusion, parenchymal infarction, and bronchial asthma. Eosinophilia often is found

FIGURE 1

Bilateral medial malleolar ankle ulcers in a patient with polyarteritis. Note the scab formation (healing) on the right.

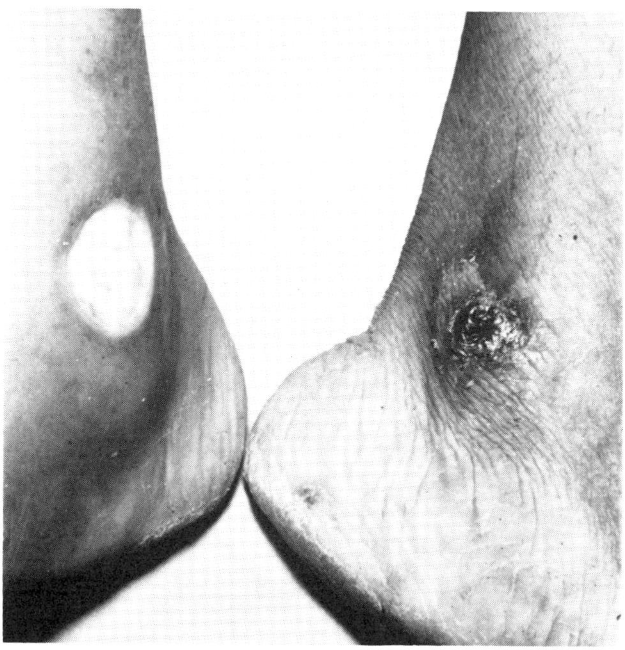

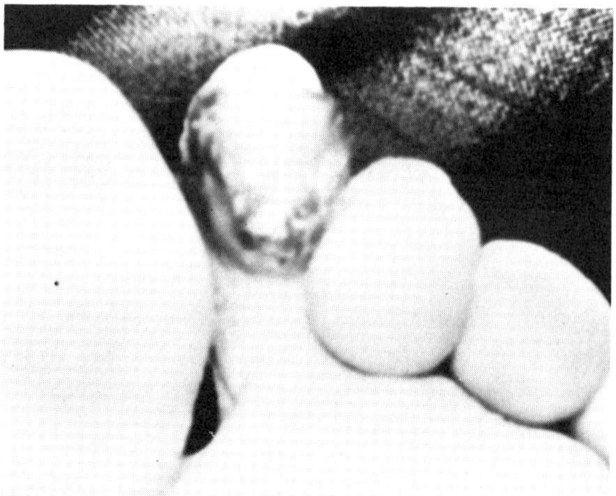

FIGURE 2
Vasculitis with early gangrenous changes of the second toe in a patient with polyarteritis.

in association with the last named. The myocardium, endocardium, pericardium, and coronary vessels may be affected. Approximately 80% of patients have central and/or peripheral nervous system involvement. Headache, seizures, and peripheral neuropathy, especially mononeuritis multiplex, are seen frequently. There may be muscle weakness, tenderness, and, later, atrophy. Joint pain is common, but inflammation is not. Arthritis may be mono- or polyarticular and frequently is migratory. Skin lesions include nodules, purpura, and gangrene. (Figs. 1 and 2).

LABORATORY TESTS

Laboratory findings are not specific: anemia, leukocytosis, eosinophilia, elevated sedimentation rate, proteinuria, and a telescoped urinary sediment are found commonly. Pulmonary infiltrates, elevated serum muscle enzymes, abnormal electromyograms and nerve conduction studies, serum HB antigen and antibody, depressed serum complement levels, and antinuclear and anti-DNA-antigens are present in selected cases. Angiography may be a valuable diagnostic aid. Characteristic findings include microaneurysms, especially at bifurcation sites; indistinct vessel outlines; segmental luminal irregularities; and obliteration and thrombosis of arteries.

DIAGNOSIS

The diagnosis of PAN is suspected clinically by the presence of a multisystem disorder, often bizarre in nature, and is confirmed histologically by the presence of arteritis. The skin, muscles, testes, and kidneys are frequent sites of biopsy (6). Typical pathologic findings include fibrinoid necrosis with a leukocytic infiltration primarily affecting the small and medium-size arteries. The leukocytic infiltration is present in and around vascular walls and is composed largely of polymorphonuclear leukocytes and frequently of eosinophils. Mononuclear cell infiltration and fibrosis occur with chronic lesions and attempts at healing. Arterial thrombosis, infarction, aneurysmal dilatation, and dissection may be found. The entire circumference of the vessel, or only part of it, may be involved; often the distribution is segmental.

COURSE AND TREATMENT

Polyarteritis usually is fatal in 6 to 12 months if untreated. Most deaths result from renal disease, with uremia and hypertension prominent features; less commonly, coronary and gastrointestinal arteritis are responsible. In some patients PAN may be limited to one or more nonvital structures, such as the skin or gallbladder, resulting in a more favorable prognosis. Other forms of vasculitis must be differentiated from PAN for prognostic and therapeutic reasons (7).

Systemic corticosteroids are helpful in many cases; in one series the 5-year survival rate approached 50%. Cytotoxic agents with or without concomitant corticosteroids improve the prognosis. Recent evidence suggests that cyclophosphamide (Cytoxan) may be the drug of choice (8).

REFERENCES

1. Talbott JH. Collagen-Vascular Diseases. New York: Grune & Stratton, 1974, p. 217.
2. Sergent JS, Lockshin MD, Christian CL, et al. Vasculitis with hepatitis B antigenemia: long-term observations in nine patients. Medicine 55:1-18, 1976.
3. Sergent JS, Christian CL. Necrotizing vasculitis after acute serous otitis media. Ann Intern Med 81:195-199, 1974.
4. Blumberg BS, Millman I, Sutnick AI, London WT. The nature of Aus-

tralia antigen and its relation to antigen-antibody complex formation. J Exp Med 134:320–329, 1971.
5. Zeek PM. Periarteritis nodosa: a critical review. Am J Clin Pathol 22:777, 1952.
6. Moskowitz RW, Baggenstoss AH, Slocumb CH. Histopathologic classification of periarteritis nodosa. Proc Mayo Clin 38:345–357, 1963.
7. Fauci AS, Haynes BF, Katz P. The spectrum of vasculitis: clinical, pathologic, immunologic, and therapeutic considerations. Ann Intern Med 89:660–676, 1978.
8. Fauci AS, Katz P, Haynes BF, et al. Cyclophosphamide therapy of severe systemic necrotizing vasculitis. N Engl J Med 301:235–238, 1979.

SCLERODERMA (PROGRESSIVE SYSTEMIC SCLEROSIS)

ROY D. ALTMAN, M.D.

Scleroderma is a descriptive term identifying a collagen vascular disease characterized by tightening of the skin. The disease is often more extensive, involving the kidney, lungs, heart, gastrointestinal tract, and skeletal muscles—hence the more accurate term of systemic sclerosis. On occasion the disease is slowly or rapidly progressive, leading to severe thickening of the skin with flexion contractures of the extremities and/or severe internal organ system involvement—hence the term progressive systemic sclerosis.

PATHOGENESIS

The etiology is unknown, but one theory involves aberrant immunity precipitating microvasculitis, particularly of the dermis. The microvasculitis precipitates edema with an inflammatory response. This sets the stage for ischemia, which stimulates fibroblastic activity. Fibroblastic stimulation precipitates excessive protocollagen and, subsequently, excessive collagen deposition. These events are most notable in the skin, but they may exist in any of the involved organ systems.

CLINICAL FEATURES

Scleroderma is present in women twice as frequently as in men, usually between the ages of 25 and 55, and is perhaps more frequent in blacks than in whites. The disease often begins with Raynaud's phenomenon or puffy swelling of the fingers that may be mistaken for rheumatoid arthritis. Raynaud's phenomenon is a frequently painful discoloration of the digits, hands, and/or feet associated with exposure of the extremity or the entire body to decreased temperature exposure. The diagnosis of Raynaud's phenomenon should involve at least two of three color phases: white (vasospasm), blue (venous stasis), red (reactive vascular dilatation of the involved or adjacent areas). Raynaud's disease may precede other aspects of scleroderma by months or years. The puffy changes of the digits often progress to the hand, with subsequent spread to the forearm, arm, face, V of the neck, lower extremities, and, perhaps, trunk. The soft puffy changes become hardened with thick atrophic skin giving a glazed, shiny appearance.

Subsequently contractures of the palmar flexors of the hand cause a "claw hand" deformity with reduced function. Sweating is decreased. Atrophic skin may have brawny hyperpigmentation with (scarred) hypopigmentation. The terminal phalanges may develop exquisitely tender ulcerated lesions along the periungual region or the distal tuft. These often heal leaving pitting scars in the skin. There may be resorption of the distal phalanx with subcutaneous calcifications that may be quite tender and painful (Fig. 1). Telangiectasias may appear on the hands and feet as well as on the face and V of the neck.

FIGURE 1

Destructive lesions of the digits with calcification in a 44-year-old female with PSS for several years.

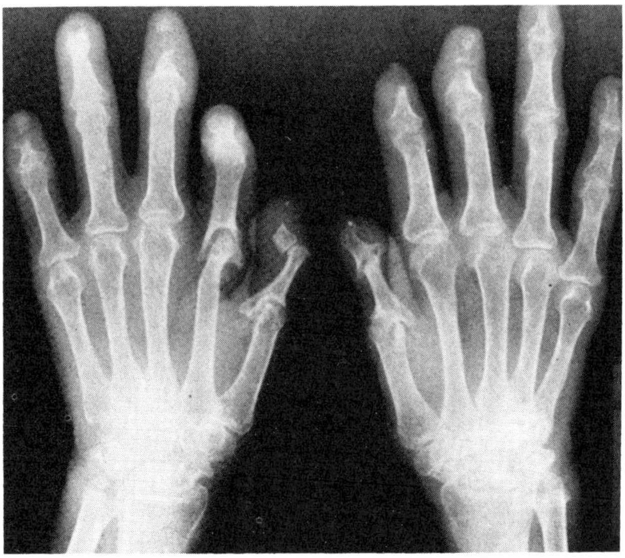

The skin of the face is at first soft and puffy with nonpitting edema. This gradually changes to thick, retracted skin. The patient loses wrinkles, particularly of the forehead on upward gaze. New wrinkles appear at the lateral corners of the eyes ("crow's feet") and about the mouth ("purse string"). The tightening about the mouth reduces the ability of the mouth to open (gape). Patients may develop Sjögren's syndrome with dryness of the eyes (keratoconjunctivitis sicca), dryness of the mouth (xerostomia), and sometimes vaginal dryness as well.

All portions of the gastrointestinal tract may be involved (Fig. 2). Dryness of the mouth leads to widening or resorption of the periodon-

FIGURE 2

Spiculation of the small bowel and reflex esophagitis caused by fibrosis and fixation of mucosal folds in a 32-year-old female with symptoms of PSS for more than a decade.

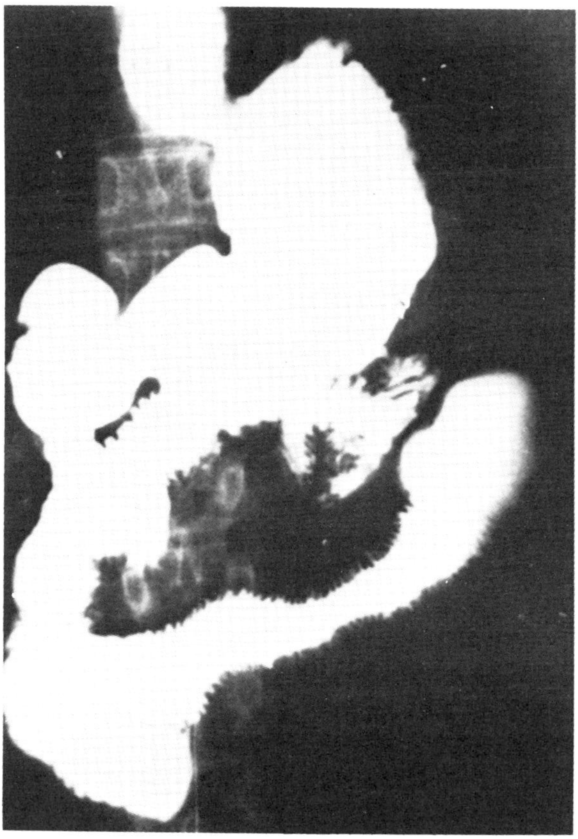

tal membrane (thinned lamina densa, Blackburn's sign). The lower esophagus and cardia of the stomach are frequently involved first with microvascular changes giving lower esophageal dysfunction with hypomotility and acid regurgitation. Lower esophageal dysphagia develops. Esophageal structure is a not uncommon complication. Reduced motility of the stomach, duodenum, and small or large bowel may develop. Dilatation of the second and third portions of the duodenum may be referred to as the "loop sign." Bowel hypomotility may allow bacterial overgrowth and a malabsorption syndrome with a megaloblastic anemia. The large bowel develops isolated areas where haustrae fail to traverse the entire bowel. This leads to usual wide-mouthed pseudodiverticulae seen on barium enema that are characteristic. Rarely, air may appear just outside the large bowel mucosa—pneumatosis cystoides intestinalis—this is an incidental radiographic finding of no clinical significance.

Joint pain may occur with active synovitis. Synovial effusions are uncommon; when present, they are relatively acellular and with good mucin clot. Tendon friction rubs may be palpated and sometimes heard under the involved skin. Atrophic muscle changes may be associated with involved skin. Occasionally muscle involvement is inflammatory and reflected by proximal muscle weakness and elevated muscle enzymes.

Cardiomegaly, pericarditis, arrhythmias, and heart failure may occur early. When present, they carry a poor prognosis. Later in the course the patient may have myocardial failure due to sclerodermatous replacement of myocardium or arrhythmias due to sclerodermatous interruption of the conduction system or secondary to pulmonary fibrosis and hypertension due to scleroderma.

Microvasculitis may involve the lungs. This potentially reversible change may respond to aggressive antiinflammatory therapy. Pulmonary involvement also portends a poor prognosis. After varying periods of time, the lungs may become fibrotic and eventually honeycombed. These later changes are not reversible and often lead to pulmonary hypertension. Esophageal dysfunction may add to this problem by facilitating aspiration. There is an increase in alveolar cell carcinoma in scleroderma. There is a suggestion of an increased incidence of scleroderma in coal miners.

Renal involvement with scleroderma almost uniformly leads to death within 6 months (Fig. 3). Occasionally death can be averted by

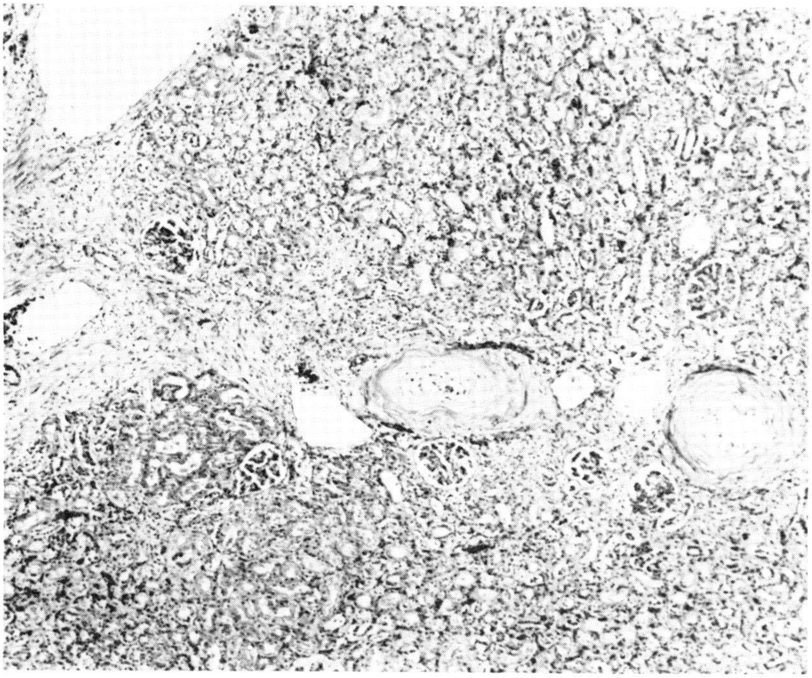

FIGURE 3

Section of the kidney taken at autopsy in a 61-year-old white female with PSS for 3 years. Concentric fibrous rings and narrowing of the lumen are seen in arteries and veins. The glomeruli and tubules appear normal.

an aggressive early and continuous therapy with antihypertensive agents. Renal scleroderma may give no warning. It often occurs within the first 2 years of disease in the edematous, progressive phase of the illness. A patient who has been relatively stable may have a premonition of impending doom within hours or days. This is followed by seizures related to severe hypertension. Renal function may be near normal upon presentation only to deteriorate slowly over the following days. Renal biopsy shows only renovascular changes compatable with essential hypertension. As renal status deteriorates, dialysis and subsequently nephrectomy-transplantation may be planned, but results are variable.

Various forms of neuritis may accompany scleroderma. Trigeminal neuralgia and diffuse pruritis are examples.

LABORATORY FINDINGS

Laboratory tests are not helpful in making the diagnosis. Hypergammaglobulineamia, hemolytic anemia (Combs' positive), elevated erythrocyte sedimentation rate, rheumatoid factor (low titer, 40%), and antinuclear antibodies (often speckled or nucleolar pattern, 20%) may be found.

COURSE

The disease course is quite variable. Death related to scleroderma is most often related to internal organ involvement such as renal, cardiac, or pulmonary disease. Most deaths occur within the first 2–3 years from the time of diagnosis. The disease tends to plateau after 2–3 years and may even show evidence of regression. There is an occasional patient who has complete or near complete resolution of the sclerodermatous skin toward normal. For unknown reasons, black patients with scleroderma have a poorer prognosis than whites.

DIAGNOSIS

Scleroderma is a clinically descriptive disease. Preliminary criteria for diagnosis have recently been published.

Major: Sclerodermatous changes proximal to the metacarpal phalangeal joints. In the absence of this criterion, two of the following three minor criteria will suffice.

Minor: Sclerodactyly: sclerodermatous changes of only the digits.
Distal digital pitting scars.
Pulmonary fibrosis.

THERAPY

No specific therapy is available that consistently prevents or retards the progressive vasculitic-fibrotic changes of this disease. Medications in the past have included such agents as paraamino benzoic acid (POTABA) and the hormone relaxin. More recent investigations suggest possible value of colchiane and D-penicillamine because both agents inhibit collagen deposition. Acute vascilitic problems of internal organs may require corticosteroids. However, their use should be restricted because there is no good evidence that prognosis is improved.

Most therapy of scleroderma is directed at the organ system involved by the sclerodermatous process. Joint symptoms may be alleviated by aspirin or NSAIDs. Physiotherapy, particularly at home, is encouraged in an attempt to retard progressive contractures. Esophageal dysfunction may be treated with "hiatus hernia regimen" including elevation of the head of the bed, small feedings, antacids, and cimetadine. Malabsorption will often respond to intermittent antibiotics. Raynaud's phenomenon does not respond to any regimen consistently. Occasional patients will respond to sympathetic blockade, peripheral blocking agents (e.g., Aldomet); however often patients benefit more from cotton gloves and reduced exposure to cold. Preliminary studies indicate that Captopril (Angiotension II enzyme inhibitor) may play a major role in therapy of renal scleroderma (5).

REFERENCES

1. Rodnan GP, chief ed. Progressive systemic sclerosis. Clin Rheum 5:49–79, 1979.
2. Altman RD. Therapy of scleroderma. Current Therapy, 1980. Philadelphia, W. B. Saunders.
3. Medsger TA Jr, Masi AT, Rodnan GP, et al. Factors affecting survivorship with system sclerosis (scleroderma): a life-table analysis of 309 patients. Ann Intern Med 75:369–376, 1971.
4. Masi AT, Rodnan GP, Medsger TA Jr, et al. Preliminary criteria for the classification of systemic sclerosis (scleroderma). Arthritis Rheum 23:581–590, 1980.
5. Lopez-Ovejero JA, Saal SD, D'Angelo WA, Cheigh JS, Stenzel KH, Laragh JH. Reversal of vascular and renal crises of scleroderma by oral angiotensin-converting-enzyme blockade. N Engl J Med 300:1417–1419, 1979.

MIXED CONNECTIVE TISSUE DISEASE

JOHN H. TALBOTT, M.D.

In recent years a distinct subset of patients combining one or more features usually considered characteristic of any one of the four unusual connective tissue disease syndromes—SLE, PSS, AD-P, and PN—for varying periods of time may be seen. Most patients eventually develop more specific features of any one of the four disorders. These observations prompted Sharp to assign to patients with overlap features the term mixed connective tissue disease (MCTD). Laboratory findings include an unusually high titer of circulating antibody to a ribonuclear protein (RNP) and usually a favorable response to corticosteroids. Almost all patients have high titers, usually greater than 1:100 and frequently greater than 1:1000 of fluorescent antinuclear antibodies of the speckled pattern type.

CLINICAL FEATURES

The majority are female. The age at development covers a wide range. Typical features include Raynaud's phenomenon, polyarthralgia or arthritis, esophageal dysfunction, inflammatory myopathy, and pulmonary disease. The appearance of Raynaud's phenomenon, swelling of the digits, and esophageal dysfunction may suggest PSS, proximal muscle weakness, AD-P, fever, arthralgias, an erythematous facial rash, dyspnea on exertion and pulmonary involvement, SLE and neurologic involvement or PN. The pathogenic process progresses slowly. Polyarthralgia occurs in most patients, with some presenting with frank nondeforming arthritis. Proximal muscle weakness may be associated with elevation of serum phosphokinase and aldolase. Muscle biopsy shows fiber degeneration and cellular infiltration. Cardiac involvement is less common than pulmonary disease, but in children it may appear as pericarditis, myocarditis with heart failure, or aortic insufficiency. Renal disease develops in a small percentage of patients but may become critical. A few show neurologic abnormalities, such as trigeminal sensory neuropathy or other types of peripheral polyneuritis. Moderate anemia or leukopenia may be present. Thrombocytopenia has been observed in children. Lymphadenopathy and Sjögren's syndrome has been reported. The characteristic serologic findings of high titers of antibody to RNP is more frequently associated with MCTD than with other rheumatic diseases. The etiology and pathogenesis are unknown.

TREATMENT AND PROGNOSIS

Mild disease may be controlled with nonsteroidal antiinflammatory drugs such as aspirin, 1–2 gm/day, or indomethacin, 50–100 mg/day, or low doses of corticosteroids, 10 to 20 mg/day. More severe symptoms require higher doses. A few have required a combination of cytotoxic drugs with or without corticosteroids. Formerly, the prognosis was thought to be somewhat better in MCTD than with any of the specifically identified connective tissue diseases. A recent follow-up of a number of patients shows that a majority progress into more typical PSS; some may develop fatal renal disease or die with SLE. Thus the prognosis should be guarded.

REFERENCES

Talbott JH, Gall EA, Consolazio WV, Coombs FS. Dermatomyositis with scleroderma, calcinosis and renal endarteritis associated with focal cortical necrosis. Arch Intern Med 63:476–496, 1939.

Sharp GC, Irvin WS, Tan EM, Gould RG, Holman HR. Mixed connective tissue disease: an apparently distinct rheumatic disease syndrome associated with a specific antibody to an extractable nuclear antigen (ENA). Am J Med 52:148–159, 1972.

Nimelstein SH, Brody S, McShane D, Holman HR. Mixed connective tissue disease: a subject evaluation of the original 25 patients. Medicine (Baltimore) 59:239–248, 1980.

EOSINOPHILIC FASCIITIS

JOHN H. TALBOTT, M.D.

What appears to be a new syndrome has been described in recent years, first by Shulman (1), followed shortly after by Rodnan and coworkers (2). Onset of symptoms develops especially in males who have recently pursued a strenuous physical life. The obvious superficial changes in the skin of the arms and legs, usually sparing the digits and the face, may suggest localized scleroderma or morphea. Others have presented with sluggish skeletal muscle movement suggestive of dermatomysitis. An orange-peel configuration of puckering of affected skin under tension is characteristic (Fig. 1). The extremities become tight; symmetrical flexion contracture of knees and elbows

FIGURE 1
Orange-peel contour of skin under tension.

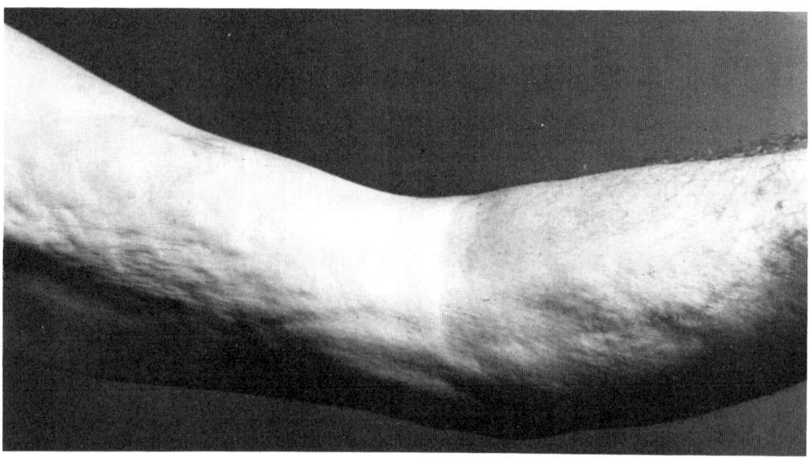

may develop. Involvement of internal organs as observed in systemic scleroderma or dermatomyositis has not been reported.

Laboratory studies have shown a negative ANA and RF. The erythrocyte sedimentation rate is elevated; sometimes the serum globulins and blood eosinophils are increased. A deep biopsy of the skin, involving subcutaneous tissue into adjacent muscle tissue showing an inflammatory reaction of the fascia, infiltrated with lymphocytes and plasma cells, and frequently with eosinophils and histiocytes, is diagnostic. Prednisone, 30–40 mg/day with rapid decrease to lower levels, 5–10 mg/day, usually is effective. Recurrences have been reported after cessation of drug therapy. Spontaneous remissions have been reported. Ultimate response awaits a longer follow-up period as isolated cases of EF with severe blood dyscrasias, autoimmune thrombocytopenia purpura, and antibody-mediated aplastic anemia have been observed.

REFERENCES

1. Shulman LE. Diffuse fasciitis with hypergammaglobulinemia and eosinophilia: A new syndrome. Presented at the VI Pan American Congress on Rheumatic Diseases, Toronto, June 16–21, 1974.
2. Rodnan GP, DiBartolomeo A, Medsger TA Jr, et al. Eosinophilic fasciitis. Report of 7 cases of a newly recognized scleroderma-like syndrome. Arthritis Rheum 18:422, 1975.
3. Talbott JH, Cusani BA. Fasciitis (eosinophilic) with scleroderma-like changes in the skin. J Fla Med Assoc 63:702–705, 1976.

POLYMYALGIA RHEUMATICA

JOHN H. TALBOTT, M.D.

Polymyalgia rheumatica is a well-defined and relatively common syndrome, occurring in older patients (+50), consisting of pain and stiffness in the proximal muscle groups without permanent weakness or atrophy. The female to male ratio is 4:1. The onset may be sudden or gradual; pain and stiffness may appear symmetrically in the neck, back, shoulder girdle, or in the pelvic girdle muscles. Morning stiffness is marked. Some patients find it difficult even to get out of bed. Fever, anorexia, malaise, weight loss, and apathy may be present. In spite of the severe pain, examination of the muscles is essentially negative. A markedly high sedimentation rate with values over 100 mm/hr, Westergren method, may be the clue to diagnosis. There may be a nonhemolytic anemia with hematocrit readings as low as 30%.

This disease is differentiated from RA by the absence of demonstrable synovitis on physical examination and a negative RF. Muscle biopsy and normal enzyme levels differentiate this from AD-P; the rapid sedimentation rate differentiates it from osteoarthritis; and normal protein electrophoresis and bone marrow differentiate it from multiple myeloma. A number of patients have an associated temporal arteritis. Irreversible blindness with headache may develop rapidly. The pathogenesis is unknown. Biopsy of an asymptomatic temporal artery may show the typical changes of giant cell arteritis. Joint scintigrams with ^{99m}technetium as pertechnetate have shown evidence of synovitis.

The disease responds in an excellent fashion to corticosteroids, which are endowed with great diagnostic as well as demonstrable therapeutic value. Treatment should be started immediately upon suspected or proven diagnosis. It should begin with 30 mg of corticosteroids daily, which is reduced promptly as symptoms subside. Corticosteroids at 5–10 mg/day levels should be continued as long as symptoms persist. In some it may be necessary to take them for many months. Salicylates, indomethacin, gold, and other nonsteroidal antiinflammatory drugs have been used in patients without proven or suspected temporal arteritis. If temporal arteritis is a probability, doses of corticosteroids as large as 60 mg/day for 1 month or longer should be taken while under the joint supervision of an ophthalmologist.

REFERENCES

1. Healey LA, Wilske KR. The Systemic Manifestations of Temporal Arteritis. New York: Grune & Stratton, 1978.
2. Fernandez-Herlihy L. Polymyalgia rheumatica. Semin Arthritis Rheum 1:236–245, 1971.

ACUTE RHEUMATIC FEVER

JOHN H. TALBOTT, M.D.

Acute rheumatic fever manifests as an inflammatory response to an infection, usually pharyngitis, by group A streptococci. Although acute migratory arthritis may be the presenting symptom, morbidity and mortality usually are associated with immediate or long-term sequelae of damage to heart muscle or heart valves. The brain (chorea), the skin (rash), and subcutaneous tissue (nodules) may be involved. Streptococcal group A organisms may be demonstrated in the acute stage of pharyngitis or, subsequently, serologically as determined by the titer of antibodies to streptococcal antigens. Recurrences and sequelae can be prevented by antimicrobial therapy of the streptococcal infection.

EPIDEMIOLOGY

ARF is commonly observed between the ages of 5 and 15 years in geographic areas with a high incidence of streptococcal disease (1). In recent decades, the incidence has decreased significantly in many countries about the world. An association with one or more specific HLA phenotype has been suggested but not proved. Patients who have had a previous attack of rheumatic fever show an increased incidence of disease from streptococcal infection, although the tendency to recurrences following infection decreases with the passage of time. Siblings may be afflicted.

PATHOGENESIS

Pathogenesis is unknown, although firm evidence shows that group A streptococci damage cardiac tissue. Although ARF cannot be produced in an experimental animal, there is some similarity between rheumatic fever and serum sickness. Serum complement, however, is decreased in serum sickness and increased in rheumatic fever. Autoantibodies to heart muscle have been found in the serum in ARF. Whether these antibodies are capable of fixing the respective antigens in vivo is uncertain. Autoantibodies to heart valves and myocardium are present in patients after cardiac surgery or with glomerulonephritis not necessarily associated with carditis. Streptococcal organisms have not been isolated from synovial fluid of clinically affected joints. There is a possibility that partly degraded streptococci or the toxins of streptococci are disseminated throughout the body. It is also possible that the arthritis of ARF may be produced by streptolysin S. Some of the streptococcal cellular constituents may be endowed with primary nonimmunogenetic toxicity.

CLINICAL FEATURES

The typical attack of ARF involves the sudden development of polyarthritis, frequently migratory, accompanied by signs and symptoms of an acute febrile illness after a latent period of from 1 to 5 weeks after a streptococcal pharyngeal infection. Large joints of the extremities are most frequently affected with an accompanying effusion. As pain and swelling subside in one joint, another joint becomes involved, sometimes within a few days. Several large joints may be involved simultaneously.

Sydenham's chorea, once a common accompaniment of ARF, is found in less than 5% of cases. The rash of rheumatic fever, erythema marginatum, is uncommon. It is a painless and evanescent erythema of the trunk and the proximal portion of the extremities, sometimes evident after a hot bath. The subcutaneous nodules of rheumatic fever are usually small, painless swellings over the bony prominences that may not be found unless searched for. There may also be epistaxis, abdominal pain, pleurisy, and a pneumonitis.

Carditis may be evident early in the disease. Organic heart murmurs, usually of mitral or aortic regurgitation or stenosis, signs and symptoms of pericarditis, and congestive heart failure may supervene. The prognosis of permanent damage is primarily related to valvular involvement.

DIAGNOSIS

Reference should be made to the Jones criteria for guidance in the diagnosis of rheumatic fever, given in the *Primer on Rheumatic Diseases*, 7th edition, 1973, which includes each of the items just noted with various degrees of significance as well as an elevated white blood cell count and presence of C-reactive protein, evidence of a proceeding B-hemolytic streptococcal infection (1).

CLINICAL COURSE

The clinical course varies greatly. The acute inflammation usually subsides within 6 weeks. Valvular lesions may heal, may remain stationary, or may undergo progressive sclerosis and calcification. There are no known criteria to predict which course the lesions will follow. With each attack the possibility of permanent damage increases. Complete subsidence of arthritis without residual joint abnormality is characterisic.

PATHOLOGY

The lesions of ARF are widely disseminated throughout the body with a special predilection for connective tissue. Local inflammatory lesions occur particularly around small blood vessels. The endocardium, myocardium, and pericardium of the heart may be involved. A submiliary granuloma, the Aschoff body, which may be seen in the myocardium, is generally considered pathognomonic. The inflammatory lesion is accompanied by swelling and fragmentation of the collagen fibers and alteration of the staining properties of the ground substance of connective tissue, known as fibrinoid degeneration. Aschoff bodies may persist for years after the rheumatic fever has been clinically quiet. They have been found in atrial appendages excised in patients operated on for mitral lesions years after the initial attack. The verrucous valvulitis of rheumatic fever leads to the most serious chronic permanent cardiac damage with varying degrees of valvular regurgitation and stenosis.

LABORATORY FINDINGS

There is an increase in antistreptolysin O titer as well as an increase in antibodies to streptococcal antigens such as antistreptokinase, antihyaluronidase, anti-DNAse, and antiNADase. The height of the antibody titer and the rate of decrement bears little relation to the severity of clinical findings. There is an increase in the erythrocyte sedimentation rate and the appearance of C reactive protein; there are also increases in serum complement, nucleoproteins, and, often, gamma globulins and fibrinogen. A prolonged PR interval frequently is found, but its appearance is an index of neither the possibility of subsequent development of rheumatic heart disease nor its severity.

TREATMENT

There is no specific cure for rheumatic fever and little that can be done, short of supportive treatment, once rheumatic fever is diagnosed. A course of penicillin should be started at once to combat the streptococci, even if throat cultures are negative. A single intramuscular injection of 1.2 million units of benzathine penicillin G or 600,000 units of procaine penicillin G intramuscular daily for 10 days should be adequate. Erythromycin is recommended for patients who are allergic to penicillin. After the completion of a therapeutic course of an antibiotic, continuous protection against a streptococcal infection should be provided.

Corticosteroids and salicylates are of great value in controlling the toxic manifestations and contribute to the comfort of the patient during acute symptoms. Salicylates are the drug of choice initially. They should be given in full therapeutic amounts, approximately 0.1 g/kg body weight ranging from 3 g in children to 6 to 8 g in adults daily, to achieve a plasma salicylate level of approximately 25 mg/100 dl. If salicylates in this dose level fail to control symptoms and signs, corticosteroids should be started, 10 to 15 mg of prednisone given four times daily. Corticosteroids are more potent than salicylates in suppressing the acute exudative inflammatory reaction. Some patients, when salicylates fail to control the disease, respond quickly to relatively large doses of corticosteroids. It is uncertain whether corticosteroids fundamentally influence the course of the disease. In severe carditis, corticosteroids seem to have no therapeutic advantage over full amounts of aspirin.

The goal of this therapy is to suppress symptoms and signs. The dosage of either drug should be reduced as improvement appears. Salicylates at subtoxic levels, 2 to 4 g/day, should be continued for several weeks; if corticosteroids are used, they should be continued at 10 to 20 mg/day for a similar period of time. If no recurrence is evident after discontinuing the drug, the attack may be considered to have been controlled. ARF should not reactivate unless a new streptococcal infection appears. The patient without carditis may resume full activity 2 months after the attack. If carditis has been present but murmurs have disappeared, full activity may be resumed after 6 months of careful observation. In patients with residual cardiac damage, the degree of damage to heart valves and myocardium usually determines future restrictions.

PREVENTION OF RECURRENCE

All patients with a diagnosis of ARF should receive interval prophylaxis indefinitely (2,3,4). Monthly intramuscular injections of 1.2 million units of benzathine penicillin G is preferred. An alternate drug is 1.0 g of sulfadiazine daily taken in a single dose or 200,000 units of potassium penicillin G twice daily on an empty stomach.

REFERENCES

1. Rodnan JP, McEwen C, Wallace SL. Primer on the rheumatic diseases. JAMA (Suppl) 224:1-152, 1973.
2. Feinstein AR, Spagnolo M, Wood HF, Taranta A, Tursky E, Kleinberg E. Rheumatic fever in children and adolescents: long-term epidemiologic study of subsequent prophylaxis, streptococcal infections, and clinical sequelae: VI. Clinical features of streptococcal and infections and rheumatic recurrences. Ann Intern Med 60(Suppl 5):68-96, 1964.
3. Kaplan EL, Bisno A, Derrick W, et al. Prevention of rheumatic fever: American Heart Association Committee Report. Circulation 55:Suppl 1-4, 1977.
4. Stollerman GH. Rheumatic Fever and Streptococcal Infection. New York: Grune & Stratton, 1975.

GONOCOCCAL ARTHRITIS

ROY D. ALTMAN, M.D.

Gonococcal (GC) arthritis is most often a complication of gonorrheal infection of the genitourinary tract and presently is the commonest form of septic arthritis. Since the advent of penicillin, most patients with GC arthritis are females in the second or third decade of life. The portal of entry for GC arthritis may be the oral or rectal mucosa, especially among homosexuals. The incidence is 1–3% of patients with gonococcal infection.

CLINICAL MANIFESTATIONS

The clinical manifestations of GC arthritis include fever, oligo- or polyarthritis, tenosynovitis, dermatitis, and, occasionally, conjunctivitis and pericarditis (1). Fever occurs in more than 50% of patients, with temperatures ranging from slightly above normal to 103° F orally. Chilliness is common, but shaking chills are not. Frequently, there is a history of migratory polyarthritis that lasts hours to days prior to settling in one or more joints. Persistently involved joints tend to be severely inflamed and exhibit marked swelling, tenderness, heat, and limitation of motion. The knee and other large joints are involved most frequently, although any peripheral joint may be affected; rarely is joint involvement symmetric. Five or more joints may be simultaneously involved with GC arthritis. Tenosynovitis may be noted during the migratory phase or subsequently and may be confused with arthritis, bursitis, or other paraarticular disorders.

A distincitve type of rash may be seen in GC septicemia and arthritis. Skin lesions are small, usually several mm in diameter, and often occur on the extensor surface of the forearm. Initially they

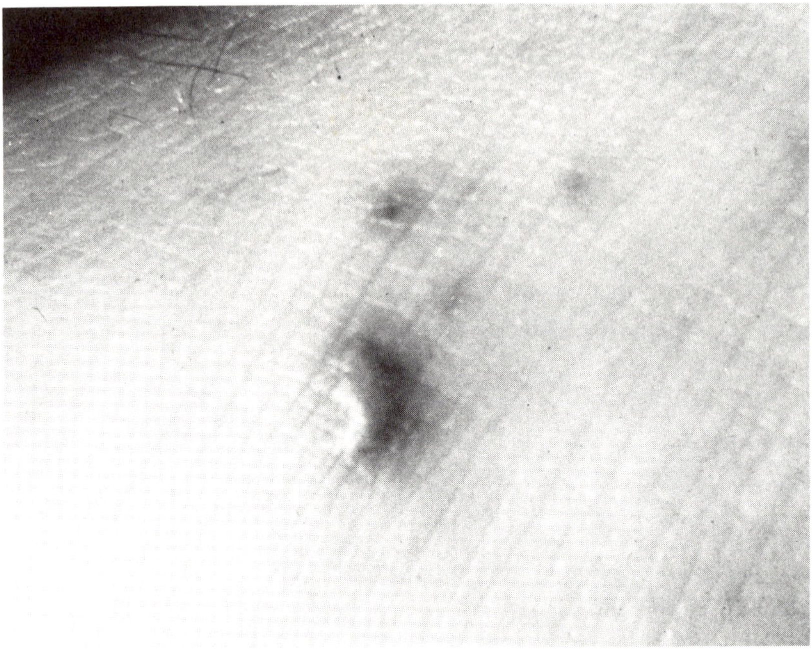

FIGURE 1
Gonococcemia: skin lesions of forearm. Lesions begin as an erythematous macule, progress to a papular, viscular, and, sometimes, hemorrhagic vesicle.

appear as an erythematous macule that then disappears or progresses to form a small vesicle or pustule. The vesicle may be hemorrhagic or have a dark necrotic center. One or several lesions that may be in different stages of development may be present (Fig. 1). Although the rash is characteristic of gonococcemia, it is not diagnostic as similar lesions may be seen with other septicemias.

There appears to be a predilection for GC arthritis during pregnancy. In fact the pregnant woman presenting with an acute arthritis must have GC arthritis considered as the first diagnosis. GC arthritis also appears to occur within a 4-day radius of the onset of the menses. However, this does not preclude GC arthritis in postmenapausal or hysterectomized women.

Immunity to gonococci is not adequate, and prior GC infections or even GC arthritis does not preclude GC arthritis.

LABORATORY FINDINGS

Laboratory tests are helpful in the confirmation of the diagnosis of GC arthritis (2). Nonspecific findings include leukocytosis, at times greater than 100,000 cells/mm^3; occasionally pronounced, elevated sedimentation rate; and the presence of intracellular gram-negative diplococci in the genital or urinary tracts.

Grossly, the synovial fluid may appear turbid or puslike; it may have a poor string sign and viscosity, an abnormal mucin precipitate consisting of polymorphonuclear leukocytes, depressed sugar, and a gram stain and synovial fluid culture that are positive for *Neisseria gonorrhoeae*. In the majority of cases, however, the gram stain and culture fail to confirm the suspected diagnosis and synovial fluid is nonspecific.

Blood, cervical, urethral, rectal, and oral pharyngeal cultures may show *Neisseria gonorrhoeae*. The pustulovesicular skin lesions may also yield gonococci. Although this organism is fragile and difficult to culture, the use of chocolate agar plates and other special media, and the immediate transfer of the culture material to the plate, increase the likelihood of growth.

X-ray changes are not ordinarily seen if diagnosis and treatment are rapid. With a delay in institution of therapy, there may be demineralization or progressive destruction of cartilage and bone with loss of normal anatomic relationships as well as occasional fibrous, or bony ankylosis.

TREATMENT

Penicillin remains the drug of choice (3). There is some controversy regarding the route and dose of penicillin, but generally doses of 1.2 million units or more of intramuscular procaine penicillin daily, in divided doses, is adequate for all but the most fulminant cases (4). With especially severe or prolonged disease, or with extraarticular manifestations of gonorrheal infection, as much as 20 million units of intravenous penicillin have been recommended. Generally, penicillin should be continued for 10 to 14 days, although some studies have suggested that treatment of shorter duration may be satisfactory, especially when massive doses of penicillin were used.

The Center for Disease Control has recommended therapy for disseminated gonococcal infection (5). The alternatives are summarized here:

1. Intravenous penicillin G, 10 million units per day in divided doses. When improvement occurs, ampicillin 0.5 gm p.o. q.i.d. to complete 7 days of therapy.
2. Tetracycline 0.5 gm p.o. q.i.d. by 7 days (avoid use in pregnant women).
3. Ampicillin 3.5 gm (or amoxicillin 3.0 gm) p.o. with probenecid 1 gm. Complete 7 day course with ampicillin (or amoxicillin) 0.5 gm p.o. q.i.d.

It is advisable to aspirate all synovial fluid at frequent intervals during therapy so as to prevent distention of soft tissues and accumulation of noxious material within the joint space (5). Rarely is surgical drainage necessary. Splinting, cold compresses, and analgesics provide symptomatic relief. Intraarticular antibiotics should not be given because they may induce an inflammatory reaction and they do not provide any additional therapeutic benefit.

The response to antibiotic therapy usually is evident within 1 to 3 days after initiation of treatment. There is a reduction in fever, joint pain, and swelling. Within 5 to 7 days little evidence of joint infection should be apparent. If treatment is delayed or inadequate, a more protracted clinical course may follow. Should cartilage or bone lesions develop, chronic degenerative arthritis of postinfectious nature may ensue.

Occasionally, patients do not respond rapidly, but have continued signs of inflammation as the synovial effusions become less cellular and more normal This type of reactive synovitis usually responds to oral nonsteroidal antiinflammatory agents.

REFERENCES

1. Brandt AS, Cathcart ES, Cohen AS. Gonococal arthritis. Arthritis Rheum 17:503–510, 1974.
2. Garcia-Kutzbach A, Dismuke SE, Masi AT. Gonococcal arthritis: clinical features and results of penicillin therapy. J. Rheumatol 1:210–221, 1974.
3. Trentham DE, McCravey JW, Masi AT. Low-dose penicillin for gonococcal arthritis: A comparative therapy trial. JAMA 236:2410–2412, 1976.
4. U.S. Department of Health, Education and Welfare, Public Health Ser-

vice, Center for Disease Control. Gonorrhea; Center for Disease Control recommended treatment schedules, 1979. Ann Intern Med 90:809-816, 1979.

5. Goldenberg DL. Treatment of septic arthritis: comparison of needle aspiration and surgery as initial mode of joint drainage. Arthritis Rheum 18:83-90, 1975.

JOINT DISEASE IN SARCOIDOSIS

JOHN H. TALBOTT, M.D.

Sarcoidosis is a disease of unknown etiology with noncaseating granulomatous involvement of various organs, which may include lungs, liver, skin, lymph nodes, eyes, and nervous tissue, as well as joints. As many as 20% of patients with sarcoidosis have articular complaints. Two patterns of involvement have been documented. A mild type of acute onset, migratory polyarthralgia or polyarthritis of peripheral joints, readily controlled; may be accompanied by fever, erythema nodosum, uveitis, and adenopathy. Large joints such as knees, ankles, and elbows tend to be involved. Symptoms may suggest periarticular inflammation as well. Radiologic examination may show only soft tissue swelling. Biopsy of the synovia shows the characteristic noncaseating granuloma.

Less often, a more persistent or chronic form of arthritis appears months or years after the onset of one or more features of nonarticular sarcoidosis. The fingers may be swollen and painful, suggesting symmetrical rheumatoid arthritis. Recurrent hydroarthrosis with joint destruction and deformity has been reported. Multiple diffuse osseous lesions, especially of the fingers, have been observed. A positive rheumatoid factor as well as a hyperuricemia and a good response to a full course of colchicine for acute symptoms may make the diagnosis more difficult. The treatment of articular symptoms is symptomatic, i.e., aspirin 1–3 gm/day or prednisone 10–20 mg/day for a short time.

REFERENCES

1. Israel HL. Joint disease in sarcoidosis. Ann Intern Med 68:1323–1326, 1968.
2. James JG, Neville E, Carstairs LS. Bone and joint sarcoidosis. Semin Arthritis Rheum 6:53–81, 1976.

PURINE METABOLISM

JULIO C. PITA, Ph.D.

The use of isotopically labeled compounds has permitted quantitative assessment of purine synthesis and degradation (1–3). As many as 50% of patients with primary gout have, in varying degrees, excessive synthesis of purines that leads to an abnormal production of uric acid (4). In some of the overproducers, as well as in the remaining group of primary gout patients, failure of renal tubular secretion of urate loads may be responsible for urate retention. In secondary gout, rapid turnover of nucleoproteins rather than the de novo pathway is responsible for hyperuricemia. In order to understand some of the biologic defects in gout, a review of the formation of adenylic and guanylic acid, purine nucleotides from which uric acid is derived, is helpful (5). Uric acid is the excreted end product of purine catabolism in human beings. The enzyme uricase, which catalyzes the oxidation of the sparingly soluble uric acid into allantoin, a more soluble substance, is absent in human beings (6).

The purine ring is formed of five carbon atoms and four nitrogen atoms. Figure 1 illustrates the origin of these atoms, which become organized in a 10-step biosynthesis sequence. The first precursor in the purine synthesis is α-D-ribose-5 phosphate from which, in a reaction depending on ATP, the α-5-phosphoribosyl-1-pyrophosphate is derived. In this reaction the pyrophosphate (PPi) group is transferred intact, producing AMP. The phosphoribosyl-pyrophosphate (PRPP) is the key intermediate in the reactions leading to the formation of purine nucleotides. In the next step, PRPP reacts with glutamine and the amino group displaces the pyrophosphate as follows:

$$\text{PRPP} + \text{glutamine} + H_2O \rightarrow \beta\text{-5-phosphoribosylamine} + \text{glutamic acid} + \text{PPi}.$$

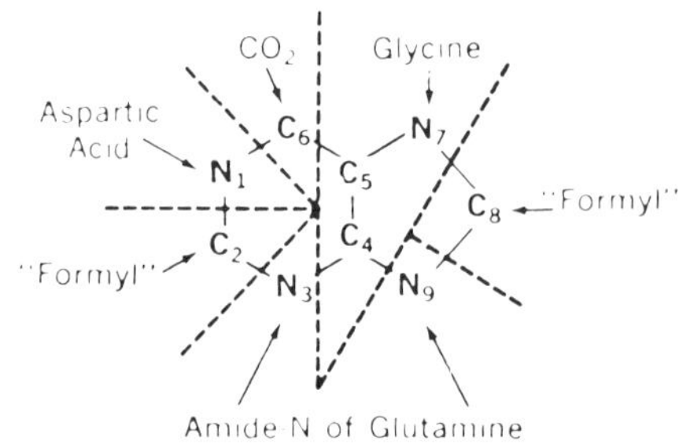

FIGURE 1
Origins of the atoms of the purine ring.

The enzyme involved in this reaction, the amidotransferase, is a multivalent regulatory enzyme that is inhibited by ATP, ADP, AMP, GTP, GDP, and GMP. Thus, as any of these mononucleotides accumulate, an early step in their synthesis undergoes a feedback inhibition. In the following step the two carbons and the nitrogen of the glycine molecule are incorporated as atoms 4, 5, and 7, respectively. The carboxyl group of the glycine reacts with the 1-amino group of 5-phosphoribosylamine in a process that also requires ATP. The product is an open-chain ribonucleotide, glycinamide ribonucleotide.

Phosphoribosylamine + glycine + ATP→glycinamide ribonucleotide + ADP + Pi

A formyl group is then donated by N^5,N^{10}-methenyltetrahydrofolate, which is a formyl group carrier, producing the following structure: P-ribose-NH-CO-CH_2-NH-CHO.

The moiety formed, α-N-formylglycinamide ribonucleotide, then receives the amide group of glutamine. This reaction requires ATP. The substance produced possesses, in open ring form, the five atoms of the imidazole portion of purine. In the ensuing reaction the chain is closed by elimination of H_2O to yield 5-aminoimidazole ribonucleotide. In the following step CO_2 is incorporated as the sixth atom in the purine ring in a carboxylation that does not require a coenzyme. The next step consists of introducing a nitrogen atom into what will become position 1 of the purine ring. An entire aspartic acid molecule is incorporated to yield 5-aminoimidazole-4-N-succinocarboxamide, from which free succinic acid is eliminated later. The last atom of the purine ring (carbon 2 in the ring) is then incorporated as a formyl group transferred from the N-formyltetrahydrofolate to the 5-amino group of the ribonucleotide. The pyrimidine portion of the purine ring is now closed with the elimination of H_2O, and the molecule of inosinic acid is completed. This is the first compound in the biosynthetic pathway with the purine ring structure. The synthesis has required five high energy phosphate bonds per mole of inosinic acid.

Inosinic acid (IMP) is the parent purine substance from which the other purine nucleotides, AMP and GMP, are synthesized. The conversion of IMP into AMP requires only the insertion of an amino group into positon 6 of the purine ring. This reaction depends on GTP and adenylsuccinate synthetase (mentioned earlier in the description of purine synthesis), which incorporates an aspartate molecule. The intermediary compound is adenylosuccinic acid. In the next step fumaric acid is released and AMP is obtained. The conversion of IMP to GMP occurs by an irreversible oxidation yielding xanthylic acid. Next, an amidation takes place in a reaction dependent on ATP with glutamine as the amino group donor. The pathway leading from inosinic to guanylic acid required ATP as a cofactor, whereas the formation of adenylic from inosinic acid requires GTP. Thus, if an excess of GMP developed, the synthesis of ATP would be accelerated; on the other hand, when there is an excess of ATP, the formation of GTP is accelerated.

This regulatory control, in addition to the feedback inhibition in the amidotransferase reaction, provides a biosynthesis regulation that maintains the formation of the mononucleotides at the molecular ratios required by the RNA and DNA complex structures. Figure 2 presents, in a schematic manner, some of these transformations. Mononucleotides result from degradation of nucleic acids by nuclease action. These compounds, adenylic and guanylic acid, undergo enzymatic partial hydrolysis losing first the phosphate group, forming the corresponding nucleosides, adenosine and guanosine. Ultimately, the free purine bases, adenine and quanine, are derived as the result of another hydrolytic step. Adenine and inosine are easily converted into uric acid via hypoxanthine→xanthine + uric acid. Guanine, losing NH_3, produces xanthine in a one-step reaction catalyzed by the enzyme guanase.

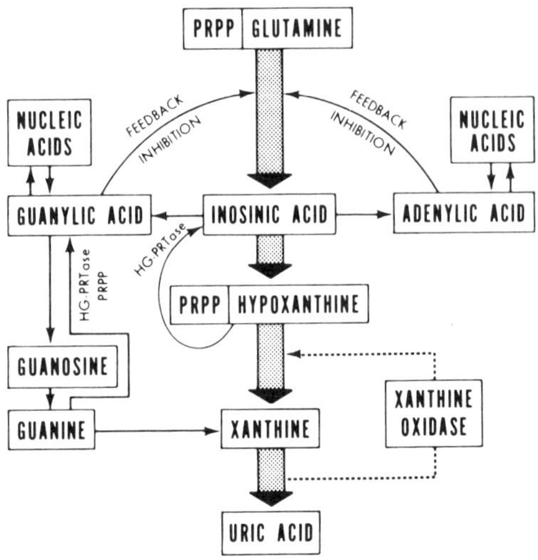

FIGURE 2

Purine nucleotides innerconversions.

The free purine bases can be salvaged and transformed again into nucleotides by at least two types of reactions:

1. Base + PRPP→nucleotide + PPi
2. Base + ribose-1-phosphate→nucleoside + Pi + nucleoside + ATP→nucleotide + ADP

The delicate balance, which includes several feedback inhibitions, normally prevents an excessive formation of uric acid. When some enzymatic deficiencies are affecting the complicated biochemical machinery, hyperuricemia may develop.

HYPERURICEMIA

Hyperuricemia accompanies glycogen storage disease, which is characterized by a deficiency of glucose-6-phosphatase. In this case two factors combine their effects. First, the patient demonstrates high plasma levels of triglycerides, lactate, and ketone bodies. Each of these substances, particularly lactate, induce a renal retention of uric acid. This impaired excretion originated by an excess of lactate has also been seen during complete fasting and in acute alcohol intoxication.

The second factor is derived from the accumulation of glucose-6-phosphate and increases the formation of α-D-ribose-5-phosphate, thus accelerating the purine synthesis.

A deficiency of the enzyme hypoxanthine-guanine phosphoribosyltransferase (HG-PRTase) occurs in children affected by the Lesch-Nyhan syndrome. Less severe deficiency has been found in other patients, all producing excessive quantities of uric acid. This enzyme catalyzes the interaction of PRPP and hypoxanthine, leading to formation of inosinic acid and, consequently, the other nucleotides derived from it. When this is deficient, hypoxanthine will accumulate and more xanthine will be produced and transformed into uric acid. In addition, more PRPP will react with glutamine, increasing the rate of purine synthesis.

Another phenomenon occurs when the enzyme amidotransferase, involved in the second step of the purine synthesis, is defective and does not respond properly to the feedback inhibitions; the control is reduced and an excessive synthesis of inosinic acid will result.

Allopurinol (Zyloprim) acts to suppress de novo synthesis or uric acid both by blocking oxidation of hypoxanthine and xanthine to uric acid and by its ribotide to inhibit the first rate-limiting step of de novo synthesis (Fig. 2).

REFERENCES

1. Lehninger AL. Biochemistry. New York: Worth, 1971, Chaps. 12 and 25.
2. Blakley RL, Vitols R. Control of nucleotide biosynthesis. Ann Rev Biochem 37:201–204, 1968.
3. Kaplan NO. Metabolic pathways involving niacin and its derivatives. In: Greenber DH, ed. Metabolic Pathways. New York: Academic Press, 1961, Vol. 2, pp. 627–672.
4. Wyngaarden JB, Kelley WN. Gout. In: Stanbury JB, Wyngaarden JB, Friedrickson DS, eds. Metabolic Basis of Inherited Disease. New York: McGraw-Hill, pp. 889–968, 1972.
5. Henderson JF. Regulation of purine biosynthesis. ACS Monograph 170. Washington, DC: American Chemical Society, 1972.
6. Kelley WN, Harris ED Jr, Ruddy S, Sledge CB. Textbook of Rheumatology. Philadelphia: W. B. Saunders, 1981, Vol. 2.

GOUT AND HYPERURICEMIA

JOHN H. TALBOTT, M.D.

Gout is primarily a disease of articular and periarticular structures caused by an increased concentration of uric acid in body fluids (1). It is one of the oldest specifically identifiable diseases, and one phase, the acute attack, responds to one of the oldest specific drugs known. Gout is the parent term. Gouty arthritis refers to joint involvement in patients with gout. The symptoms of acute gouty arthritis are associated with the presence of sodium urate crystals in synovial fluid and probably their phagocytosis by leukocytes. A persistent bona fide elevation of the serum uric acid is the sine qua non of gout. Hyperuricemia may be caused by a single aberration of normal metabolism or by a combination. This multiple concept of pathogenesis suggests the polygenic origin of gouty arthritis, although the clinical findings and therapeutic responses are indistinguishable at this stage of our knowledge.

Primary gout is the term applicable to symptoms and hyperuricemia that are the result of a heritable disorder of purine biosynthesis (see the previous chapter on Purine Metabolism) leading to the overproduction of uric acid, or a heritable dysfunction of the renal exchange of uric acid, or, in some patients, a combination of causes (2). As a heritable disorder a significant familial incidence of clinical gout as well as an increased prevalence of hyperuricemia in close relatives of gouty patients is well documented. In addition to familial or primary gout, there are a few uncommon disorders in which the basis of genetically determined hyperuricemia has been identified (e.g., Lesch-Nyhan syndrome, glycogen storage disease type I) (3).

The term secondary gout refers to symptoms similar to primary gout, but the hyperuricemia is caused by an increased turnover of nucleoproteins or a disturbance of renal transport of uric acid, clearly identified in each category. Examples include hemolytic disorders, such as polycythemia or myelofibrosis; the altered renal excretion of uric acid following thiazide ingestion; and saturnine gout, which follows chronic lead poisoning (4).

CLINICAL FEATURES

Approximately 95% of patients with primary gout are males. The initial articular episode usually appears in the fourth or fifth decade of life. Gout has been reported, but is rare, in prepubertal males. Its onset has been recorded as late as the ninth decade of life.

The usual initial feature of gouty arthritis is the appearance of an acute arthritic attack, sudden in onset, in a peripheral joint without warning, in a middle-aged male. The arthritis may be monoarticular or polyarticular. The great toe is involved in more than 50% of the initial episodes (Fig. 1) and in most patients one or more times, in the natural course of the disease. Hence, the traditional term, podagra, frequently used and assumed by some to be synonymous with gout.

FIGURE 1

Anteroposterior view of feet of a 76-year-old black female with a 6-year history of arthritis. Serum uric acid was elevated. The acute attacks responded to full courses of colchicine.

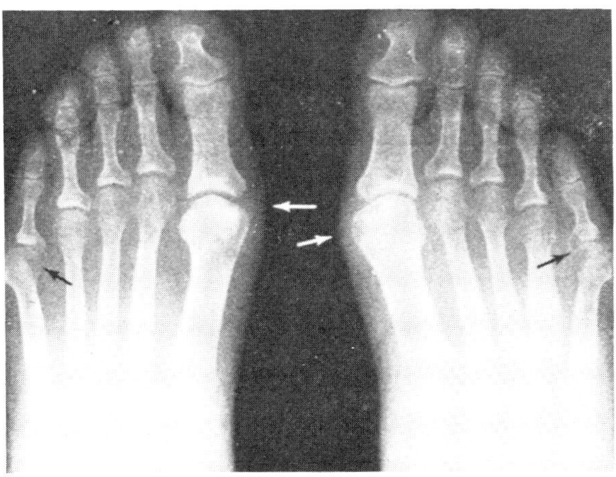

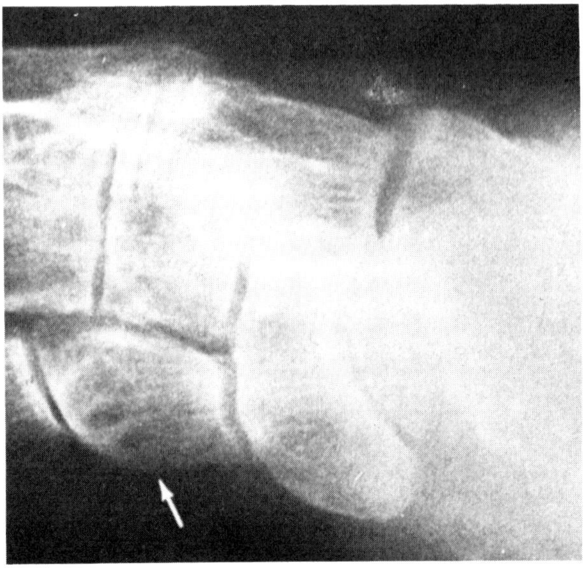

FIGURE 2

Anteroposterior view of right foot with multiple cystic lesions in an 83-year-old black female with a long history of gouty arthritis. The patient responded well to full courses of colchicine.

Other joints affected during the acute attack or later with tophaceous deposits, in order of involvement, include ankle (Fig. 2), knee, hand, wrist, and elbow. The hip and shoulder are involved rarely. In only a few cases have tophi been observed in the intervertebral, sacroiliac, or sternoclavicular joints. If the hyperuricemia persists uncontrolled for years or decades, tophi appear within or around affected joints and eventually a state identified as chronic tophaceous gout appears.

PRECIPITATING AGENTS

Acute attacks may be precipitated by a variety of agents. These include excessive use of a particular type of alcoholic beverage, sexual debauchery, a high purine meal, an acute infection, a minor or major surgical operation, physical or emotional trauma, or a number of drugs including penicillin, thiamine, and mercurial or other diuretics.

LABORATORY FINDINGS

The serum uric acid concentration usually is increased if the serum is sampled when the patient has abstained from hypouricemic drugs for several days. In most gouty patients it varies between 8 and 10 mg/100 dl; in a few it may be as high as 12 or 14 mg/100 dl. There may be considerable variation in the values based upon the method of measurement; the automated procedure usually has an upper limit of normal of 8 or 8.5 mg/100 dl. The upper limit for adult females is approximately 1 mg/100 dl less than males.

IDIOPATHIC HYPERURICEMIA

With the gross proliferation of comprehensive determinations of chemical constituents in the adult population, as many as 10% of adult males will have an unexplained (idiopathic) hyperuricemia without

FIGURE 3
Tophaceous gout in a 56-year-old male who suffered from arthritis for at least 15 years.

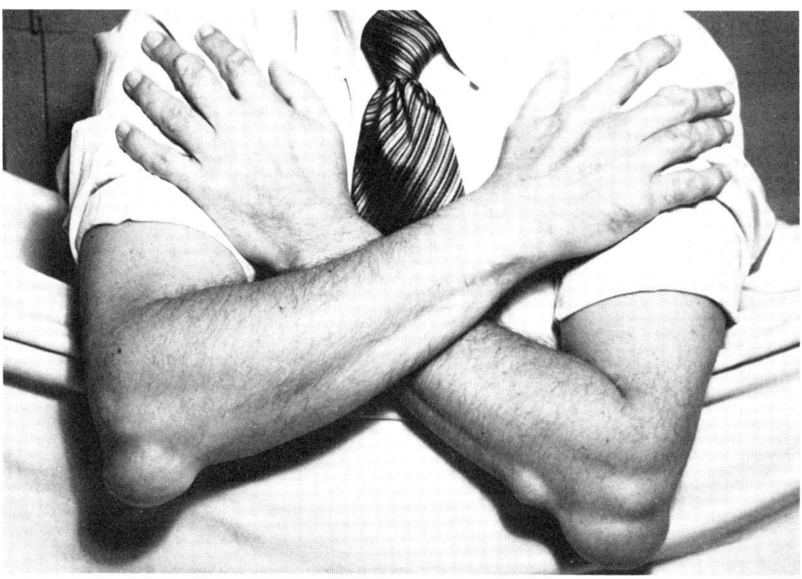

articular symptoms. The probability of an acute attack of gout developing in any decade in a male with idiopathic hyperuricemia is slight.

SEVERE CHRONIC TOPHACEOUS GOUT

Severe chronic tophaceous gout is the fate of only a small percentage of patients, particularly those who have not had the benefit of potent antigout drugs. The urate deposits may be evident on subcutaneous palpation about the joints of the toes, hands, and, less often, elbows and knees, or radiographically as small erosions in the subchondral areas of the joints of the hands or the feet.

Tophi are rarely seen at the time of the initial attack and may never appear with adequate antigout therapy. In chronic tophaceous gout (Fig. 3) the skin over a long-standing tophus may break down and a sinus may form with oozing of urate sludge.

DIAGNOSIS

There are four primary criteria for a diagnosis of acute gouty arthritis. All four may be satisfied in many patients, three in most patients, and rarely two criteria (2 and 3) may suffice. These four criteria are:

1. The development of an acute attack, sudden in appearance and severe in nature, of a peripheral joint, usually in a male in the middle decades of life, associated with the cardinal signs of inflammation (i.e., heat, redness, tenderness, and swelling). The symptoms may subside spontaneously after several days or more rapidly with specific antigout drugs. Between attacks early in the clinical course or later if adequately treated, the joints are normal subjectively and objectively upon inspection.
2. The identification of uric acid crystals in synovial fluid. Sometimes these may be engulfed by phagocytes; at other times they are floating free in the fluid (Fig. 4).
3. The therapeutic response to a full course of colchicine. This usually consists of 4 to 6 mg of colchicine given orally in divided doses without interruption over a period varying from 8 to 12 hr. Beginning improvement should be noted at the end of this course. Sig-

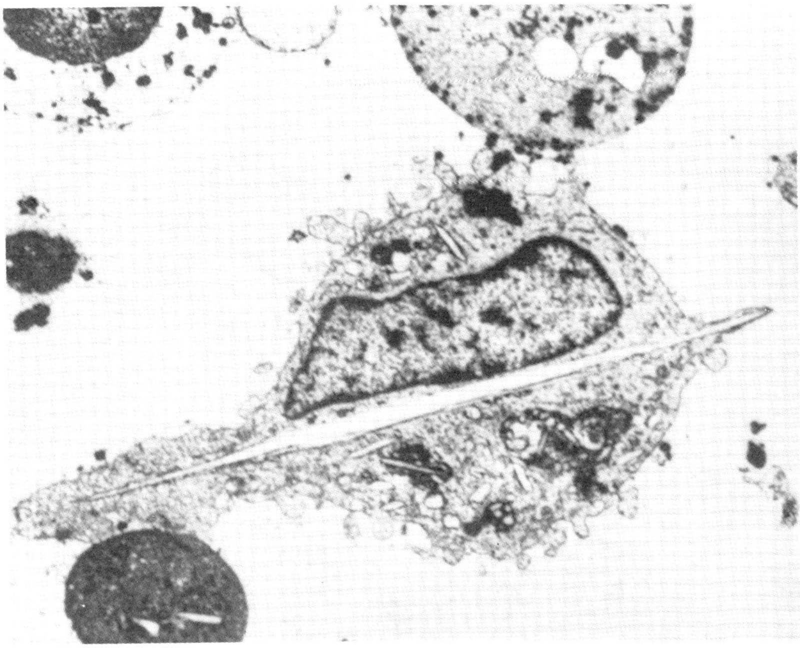

FIGURE 4
Engulfed urate crystal in leukocyte.

nificant improvement should be observed 12 to 18 hr later. Subsidence of most distress in 36 to 48 hr should be expected.

4. A persistent elevation of serum uric acid. It is a common practice for patients with unexplained joint pain, sudden in onset, to take a medicine cabinet analgesic such as one containing salicylates, which will lower the uric acid level in the serum. If the patient has hyperuricemia, a few tablets taken as self-medication may depress an otherwise elevated level into the normal range. If the uric acid concentration is normal, and the symptoms are highly suggestive of gout, the uric acid determination should be repeated after the patient has abstained for several days from all drugs that influence the uric acid level. Usually it is not advisable to take the patient off drugs immediately after the acute attack because of the danger of a recurrence. It is permissible to wait several weeks before taking the patient off all drugs that affect uric acid values in order to repeat the serum uric acid determination.

A 24-hr urine specimen should also be collected to determine the content of uric acid. From 500 to 700 mg is a normal amount of uric acid for this period. Knowledge of the 24-hr urinary output of uric acid may be helpful in directing therapy. Either a low output, less than 400 mg, or an increasingly high output, more than 1000 mg, suggests the use of allopurinol as the uric acid drug of choice. In the majority of patients, either probenecid or allopurinol may be used as a uric acid prophylactic drug, together with colchicine, each taken daily.

X-rays taken at the time of the first attack, or at some time after, are essentially normal except for soft tissue swelling. Osseous or subcutaneous tophi are late manifestations and may not appear for several years after the first attack, and, in many patients, will never appear if antigout therapy is continuous and adequate.

COURSE

At the time of the first attack it is folly to predict the long-range course of primary gout in any patient. If the initial symptoms appear in the fifth or sixth decade of life and the uric acid is in the moderate gouty range only, the patient may have the disease in a mild form and will never progress into the chronic tophaceous stage, even without the drugs that influence uric acid metabolism. At the other end of the scale is the young person who develops symptoms early in life, such as in the third decade, with a marked elevation of serum uric acid. Since the disease is progressive, without daily prophylactic therapy it may advance into the chronic tophaceous stage within a decade. Intermediate between these extremes is the patient with moderate gout who suffers the initial attack in the third or fourth decade, has no serious complications, follows the prescribed regimen carefully, and thereby avoids the development of chronic tophaceous changes. Such a patient has little or no distress because of prevention of recurrences of acute articular attacks through proper therapy. The person is able to live an essentially normal life in all major respects.

COMPLICATIONS

A number of patients with gout, as many as 20%, pass one or more renal stones per decade, usually at infrequent intervals. In only a few patients is more than one stone passed per year. Urate stones are characteristically small and range in color from pale yellow to black. Some may contain detectable amounts of calcium.

A number of gouty patients will have an elevation of blood pressure, transient or persistent, usually systolic, although a mild elevation of the diastolic pressure is not unusual. A number of patients, and not always the same oncs, will show persistent or transient albuminuria.

Less than 10% of patients with gout will die prematurely from a disease-related complication. Renal insufficiency is the usual cause. Whether adequate prophylactic therapy will reduce the incidence of serious renal disease, decade by decade, remains to be determined. However, there is cause for optimism. There is no evidence at present that this may be true for probenecid or allopurinol, although no statistical evaluation of this function has been made in any large series of patients.

TREATMENT

Specific indications for treatment are highly successful when followed and sadly disappointing when ignored. The approach to specific therapy is twofold and is an excellent example of indispensable polypharmacy. The disturbance of uric acid metabolism must be treated simultaneously with the use of colchicine, which prevents recurrences of acute articular distress.

Colchicine has been identified for more than 200 years as a specific chemical compound. Its active principle has been recognized empirically as an antigout drug for many more centuries. Colchicine has no specific effect upon uric acid metabolism or consistently upon any type of joint disease other than gout. Furthermore, it is highly specific in the treatment of the acute attack of gouty arthritis when properly given, and it is highly efficient in preventing recurrences when taken daily in a long-range prophylactic regimen. For the treatment of the acute attack, a full course is indicated. One mg should be taken orally every 2 hr until the onset of gastrointestinal distress or significant relief of symptoms, whichever occurs first. Colchicine is then stopped. If gastrointestinal distress has appeared, this side effect is handled with tincture of camphorated opium, 5 dl every three stools. Colchicine is not resumed until several days have elapsed. Intravenous colchicine may be substituted for oral colchicine. It is effective in somewhat smaller doses, 2 mg each dose every 4 hours, and is not associated with gastrointestinal symptoms. During the intercritical period, as a prophylactic agent, from 0.5 to 1.5 mg of colchicine should be taken daily depending upon whether the disease is mild, moderate, or severe. Until further evidence is available, colchicine should be continued year after year. The only untoward effect of daily colchicine is a self-limited gastrointestinal irritation when the dose exceeds tolerance.

The disturbance of uric acid metabolism is amenable to correction by two different groups of pharmacologic agents. These agents are either uricosuric or enzyme inhibiting. Probenecid (Benemid) has been available for three decades as an effective uricosuric agent. It has no basic effect upon involved joints. However, it exerts a secondary effect upon such joints. This is associated with the inhibition of further deposition of urates and the lowering of the body pool of uric acid, which withdraws urates from the joints. The pharmacologic action of probenecid is exerted upon the renal transport of uric acid, causing a significant increase in uric acid excretion. This action holds for normals as well as gouty patients. The dose varies from 0.5 to 1.5 gm per day, depending upon the severity of the gout. It should be taken at meals. A small percentage of patients develop gastroirritability to probenecid, which may be controlled with antacids or by ingestion with food. A few patients show a hypersensitivity reaction that, if not controlled with antihistaminics, should signal the use of another agent.

Allopurinol (Zyloprim) is the second type of agent that affects uric acid. It decreases the formation of uric acid by inhibiting xanthine oxidase. An enzyme that has been available for a decade and a half, it shows a slightly higher index of toxicity than does probenecid. Sometimes this is no more than gastrointestinal irritability, less often the more serious development of exfoliative dermatitis. If such a sequence of events follows, the patient should not be rechallenged with the drug. The dose varies from 200 to 600 mg a day depending upon severity.

In patients with moderate or severe tophaceous gout, the three antigout drugs—colchicine, probenecid, and allopurinol—should be given continuously day after day. If hypersensitivity does not develop, they may be continued year after year. Failure in the control of symptoms can usually be attributed to a lack of understanding of the pharmacology of the antigout drugs by the physician or need for daily compliance by the patient.

A chronic stone former, a patient who has hyperuricemia in the high gouty range, or one who exceeds 1000 mg of uric acid daily should benefit from a restricted purine intake and daily allopurinol. Foodstuffs high in purines such as kidneys, liver, sweetbreads, sardines, and anchovies are contraindicated. Most patients with gout who take the antigout drugs regularly may eat a normal diet otherwise; alcoholic beverages are not prohibited unless they can be shown to induce acute exacerbations. A high fluid intake is important because of the limited solubility of sodium urate in body fluids, including the fluids that transport uric acid through the kidney. An obese patient should lose weight as in other types of arthritis. Large, persistent tophi, usually about the elbow, knee, or Achilles tendon, should be removed surgically. If chronic tophaceous changes have deformed the hands, plastic surgery is recommended similar to corrective surgery in chronic deforming RA.

Once the diagnosis has been made, a full course of colchicine may not be needed in the recurrence of an acute attack. If the patient is on daily prophylaxis, however, the incidence of recurrences is insignificant. As a substitute for colchicine, sulindac (Clinonil) 400 mg a day, or indomethacin, 100 to 200 mg a day for 2 or 3 days, are proper choices. There is no place for corticosteroids in the treatment of acute or chronic gouty arthritis, except for unusual circumstances when large amounts of ACTH gel have been found to be effective, 60 to 80 units intramuscularly for 1 or 2 days.

ASYMPTOMATIC HYPERURICEMIA

Asymptomatic hyperuricemia should be treated only if the hyperuricemia is in the high range, as a persistent finding, such as over 10 mg/100 dl, and the hyperuricemia appears early in life, such as in the second decade. Most patients with idiopathic hyperuricemia should not be placed on any prophylactic regimen until after the onset of acute gouty arthritis. The chance of this developing is slight. If it does appear, symptoms can be adequately handled as in primary gout. Time has not run out in this case. Nor has it been shown that irreversible damage has been done to kidneys or blood vessels while withholding medication. Until further indications warrant prophylactic therapy, a conservative course of action is justified.

REFERENCES

1. Talbott JH, Yü TF. Gout and Uric Acid Metabolism. New York: Stratton Intercontinental, 1976.
2. Rieselbach RE, Sorensen LB, Shelp WD, Steele TH. Diminished renal urate secretion per nephron as a basis for primary gout. Ann Intern Med 73:359-366, 1970.
3. Lesch M, Nyhan WL. A familial disorder of uric acid metabolism and central nervous system function. Am J Med 36:561-570, 1964.
4. Ball GV, Sorensen LB. Pathogenesis of hyperuricemia in saturnine gout. N Engl J Med 280:1199-1202, 1969.
5. Wallace SL. Colchicine. Semin Arthritis Rheum 3:369-381, 1974.

PATHOPHYSIOLOGY OF CARTILAGE

J. F. WOESSNER, Jr., Ph.D

Articular hyaline cartilage is a connective tissue especially adapted to undergo continuously changing forces of compression. This type of cartilage consists chiefly of large hydrophilic aggregates of chondromucoprotein (proteoglycan) held in place by a three-dimensional meshwork of collagen fibers. Scattered through this extracellular matrix are small islands occupied by chondrocytes, the cells responsible for the synthesis and maintenance of the extracellular collagen and proteoglycan molecules. There is little blood supply to the cartilage so that the nutrition of the chondrocytes depends to a large extent on the diffusion of nutrients and oxygen through the matrix.

PROTEOGLYCAN

The structure of cartilage proteoglycan is illustrated in Figure 1. Although most of this information is derived from a study of bovine nasal cartilage, there is good reason to believe that human articular cartilage proteoglycans are similar (1). The basic building block of the proteoglycan is the proteoglycan monomer. This consists of a long protein chain that serves as a core for the attachment of polysaccharide side chains. Two types of side chains are intermingled along the core: chondroitin-6-sulfate, made up of alternating molecules of glucuronic acid and N-acetyl-galacto-samine-6-sulfate; and keratan sulfate, composed of alternating galactose and N-acetyl-glucosamine-6-sulfate or galactose-6-sulfate. These polymers of sugar and uronic acid have molecular weights (MW) of about 20,000 daltons. Since the whole subunit weighs about 2,000,000 daltons, there must be approximately 100 such chains distributed along the protein core.

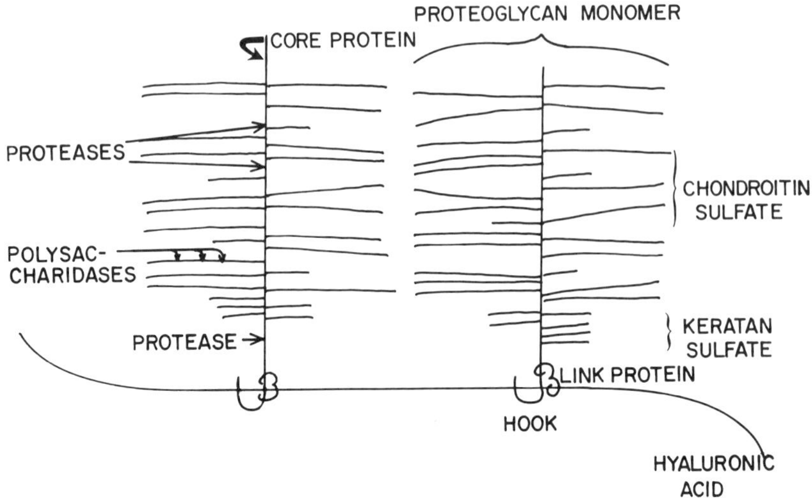

FIGURE 1

Structure of the proteoglycan aggregate of cartilage.

The keratan sulfate chains are thought to be predominantly clustered near the linkage end of the core. All the chains are negatively charged, so there is a tendency for mutual repulsion leading to a structure similar to a bottle brush.

The monomers can become aggregated to large aggregates weighing about 30,000,000 daltons. The individual monomers bind onto a chain of hyaluronic acid, which is composed of alternating glucuronic acid and N-acetyl-glucosamine residues. One end of the core protein is modified for this purpose and is free of side chains in the link region. However, an auxiliary glycoprotein or link protein is required to stabilize the union of monomer with the hyaluronic acid chain.

The negative charges from the sulfate ions render the proteoglycan aggregate strongly anionic. One effect of this charge is that the aggregate becomes maximally extended, permitting it to hold large amounts of water. Pathologic breakdown of the aggregate leads to loss of water-holding capacity. The aggregate also binds ions with positive charges; in particular there is usually considerable bound calcium. The matrix can be stained with cationic dyes such as safranin O.

Pathologic breakdown of the proteoglycan aggregate occurs in various diseases, especially osteoarthritis and rheumatoid arthritis. Such breakdown is one of the early steps in these diseases; collagen breakdown probably occurs secondarily. One way to produce breakdown is through the action of enzymes that cleave sugar chains. Hyaluronidase, an enzyme found in human testes and liver, will digest both the hyaluronic acid thread that holds the aggregate together and the chondroitin and keratan sulfate side chains of the monomer. Digestion of the hyaluronic acid chain would liberate monomers of 2,000,000 daltons, but these would be too large to move through the thicket of neighboring molecules and could not escape from the matrix. On the other hand, considerable activity of hyaluronidase would be required to digest all the polysaccharide side chains of the monomer. Moreover, it has not been possible to demonstrate hyaluronidase activity in articular cartilage.

However, there are a number of proteolytic enzymes in the cartilage. These proteases are able to digest the protein core or backbone of the aggregate. This would liberate small clusters of polysaccharide chains attached to peptide fragments. Such clusters of 20,000 to 100,000 daltons could then diffuse from the tissue and eventually be carried off in the circulation or further digested inside the chondrocyte.

The chondrocytes contain packets of hydrolytic enzymes, i.e., lysosomes. One can produce arthritis models by injecting agents such as filipin or vitamin A into the knee joint. This causes the cells to discharge their lysosomal enzymes into the extracellular matrix. This is rapidly followed by depletion of the proteoglycans, leaving behind an empty collagen meshwork and a severely damaged joint.

The most prominent proteolytic enzyme in the articular cartilage is cathepsin D. This enzyme is closely related to pepsin, and, like pepsin, requires an acid pH (about 4 to 5) to function. Cathepsin D is elevated in human cartilage in arthritis. However, it does not digest proteoglycan aggregate in the pH range of 6 to 7.5, and it is unlikely that this enzyme is responsible for damage to the extracellular matrix. The cartilage also contains one or more proteases that can digest aggregate at physiologic pH. These low molecular weight metalloproteases may be responsible for the loss of matrix seen in osteoarthritis (2). Similar enzymes may be released into the joint by leukocytes in rheumatoid arthritis, causing severe and rapid destruction.

COLLAGEN

The second major component of cartilage is the fibrous protein, collagen. The synthesis and assembly of collagen are illustrated in Figure 2. Many changes are introduced in the collagen molecule after synthesis of the protein takes place (3). First, certain residues of proline and lysine are oxidized by special hydroxylases to form the unusual amino acids, hydroxyproline and hydroxylysine. Hydroxyproline is

FIGURE 2
The pathway of collagen synthesis.

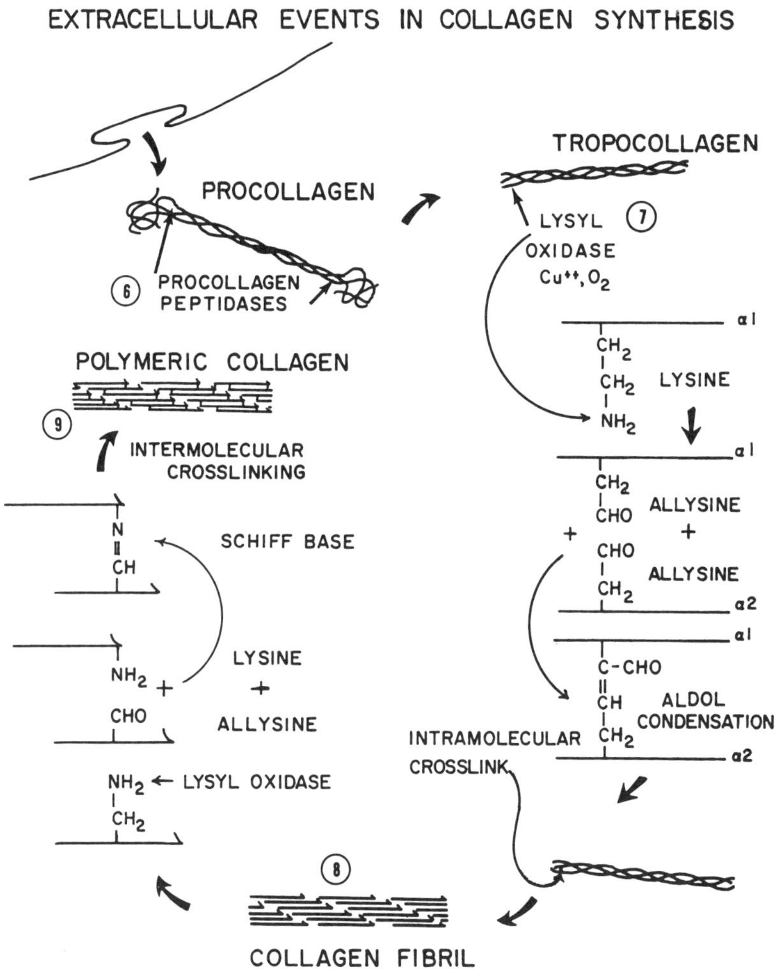

needed to stabilize the triple-helical structure of the collagen molecule; otherwise this structure would collapse at body temperature. Hydroxylysine serves as a point of attachment for galactose and glucosyl-galactose. Without these sugars, the collagen molecule cannot be properly transported from the cell into the extracellular space.

FIGURE 2 *(continued)*

INTRACELLULAR EVENTS IN COLLAGEN SYNTHESIS

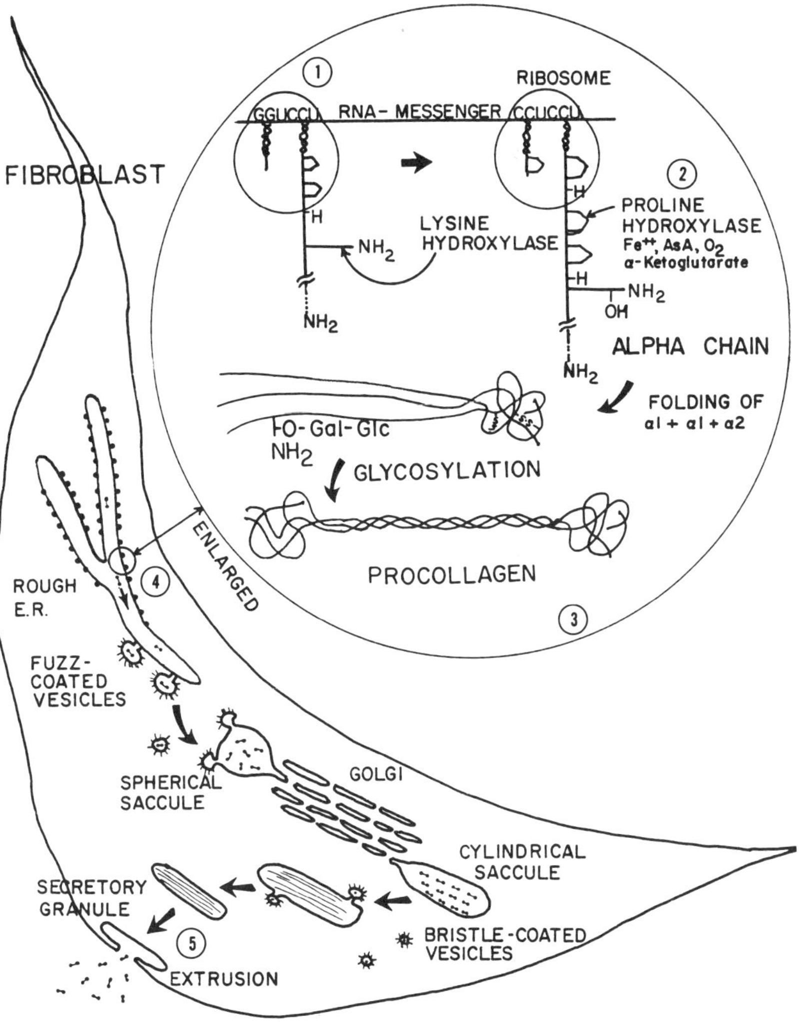

Another event occurring in the cell is the folding into the triple helix. This requires the coming together of three alpha chains of procollagen in correct alignment. Such alignment is produced by the prior folding of the carboxy-terminal portions of alpha chains and the forming of disulfide bridges. When this folding is complete, the remaining portions of the alpha chains twist around each other to form the triple helix. The ability to form such helices resides in the special feature of the alpha chains that they have the smallest amino acid, glycine, in every third position along the chain.

When the molecule has been folded and glycosylated, it migrates to the extracellular space. Here it encounters peptidases that clip off the registration peptides, converting procollagen to tropocollagen. When molecules of tropocollagen collide, they tend to hold together and to align themselves into long filamentous arrays or microfibrils. These microfibrils grow until they are 5 molecules in cross section and thousands of molecules in length. The molecules form staggered arrays by clinging to other molecules lying alongside. The head of one molecule never makes contact with the tail of the molecule in front of it; rather there is always a gap. The microfibrils are collected into larger bundles called fibrils. These are the structures commonly seen in the electron microscope and readily identified by their highly regular pattern of crossbands repeated every 670 Å.

The final event in the history of collagen formation is the development of cross-links between adjacent molecules. An enzyme, lysyl oxidase, converts certain lysine molecules near the two ends of each molecule into allysine, i.e., a lysine with an aldehyde group. Two aldehydes or an aldehyde and amino group on neighboring protein molecules can interact to form covalent crosslinks as illustrated.

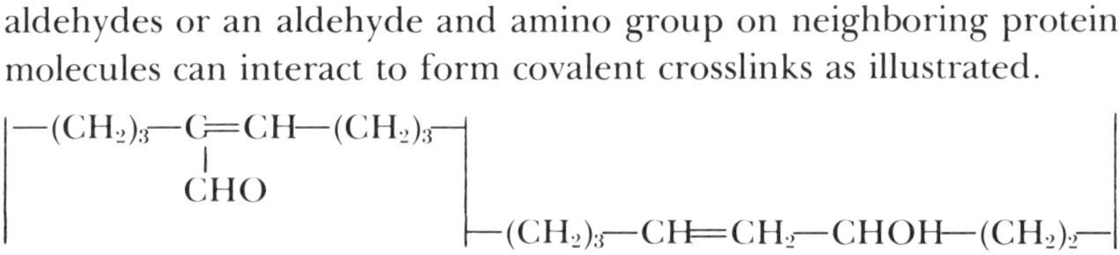

Until this cross-linking occurs, the collagen fibrils have no strength and can easily be stretched and torn.

It is apparent that many separate steps are required to produce a functioning collagen fibril. If something can go wrong, it usually will. Indeed, defects and diseases are recognized for each of the steps outlined. However, most of these known pathologies are not manifested in the cartilage or are not prominent. On the other hand, a number of pathologic changes in cartilage involve the breakdown of collagen.

A scheme of such collagen breakdown is illustrated in Figure 3. In cartilage, the collagen probably must be denuded of enveloping proteoglycan before it is susceptible to degradation (4,5). The exposed fibers are termed polymeric collagen because of the extensive cross-linking of collagen. The polymeric collagen fibers, as well as individual tropocollagen molecules, are digested by a specific collagenase. This enzyme cuts across all three alpha chains of collagen at a point one-quarter of the molecular length from the C-terminus. The two fragments of collagen then lose their helical structure at 37° and can be further digested by other nonspecific proteases. In some tissues

FIGURE 3
Pathways for the breakdown of collagen.

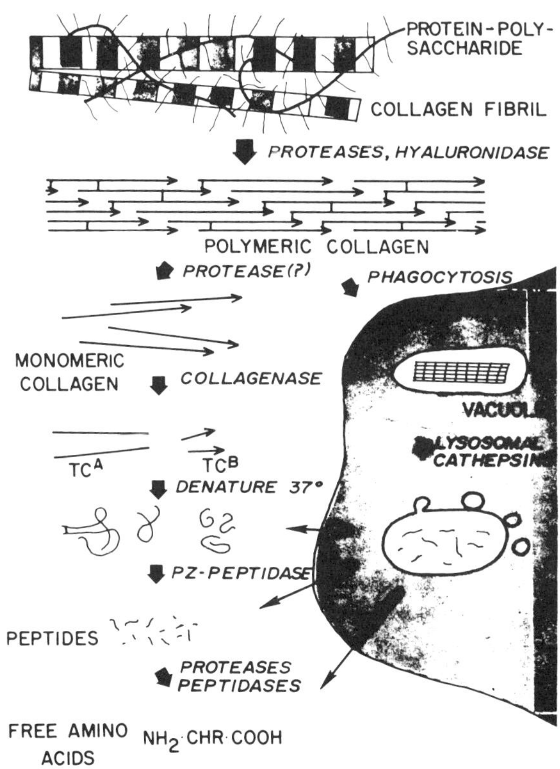

where collagen breakdown is extremely rapid, collagen fibrils are phagocytosed by cells and digested by lysosomal enzymes. There is evidence for such phagocytosis in rheumatoid arthritis. The cartilage matrix has recently been shown to contain collagenase in osteoarthritis. In rheumatoid arthritis collagenase is produced by modified synovial membranes and by leukocytes. It is released into the synovial fluid and makes its way to the cartilage. There is also rich secretion by the pannus into the underlying matrix. This protease then completes the destruction of the extracellular matrix that was begun by the digestion of the proteoglycan.

UNIQUENESS OF CARTILAGE MATRIX

Recent evidence demonstrates the existence of two distinct species of collagen produced by two distinct genes. Bone and skin contain type I collagen; cartilage contains type II collagen. Type II collagen contains much more hydroxylysine than does type I; most of these residues have sugar molecules attached to them. Type II collagen cannot be calcified to form bone. To convert cartilage to bone, the extracellular matrix must be completely replaced by a new matrix of different composition. The well-known tidemark separating bone from articular cartilage is now seen as the dividing line between two completely different types of collagen. It is further known that when the articular cartilage is damaged, or a portion is excised, the repair is performed by fibroblastlike cells that produce type I collagen. This means that normal cartilage will never be established in the damaged area and joint function may eventually be lost (3).

A further feature of cartilage structure is that the chondrocyte forms around itself a special region known as its territory and it secretes a special matrix, the territorial matrix, as a nest surrounding itself. This territorial matrix is different from the major portion of the cartilage matrix. It consists of a basketwork of type I collagen filled with hyaluronic acid and rich in lysozyme.

ADDENDUM

An International Symposium was held October 1–3, 1980, in Palm-Aire, Florida. Approximately 80 contributions were presented discussing some of the most recent findings regarding the Inflammatory

Component in the Pathology of Osteoarthritis. These included discussions on cartilage proteoglycans, articular collagen, synovial and cartilage enzymes, cellular and humoral factors, cartilage inflammation and specific drugs in osteoarthritis. The Proceedings will appear as a Supplement in Seminars in Arthritis and Rheumatism 10:231-379, 1981.

REFERENCES

1. Heinegard D, Hascall VC. Aggregation of cartilage proteoglycans. J Biol Chem 249:4250-4256, 1974.
2. Sapolsky AI, Howell DS, Woessner JF Jr. Neutral proteases and cathepsin D in human articular cartilage. J Clin Invest 53:1044-1053, 1974.
3. Nimni ME. Collagen: its structure and function in normal and pathological connective tissues. Semin Arthritis Rheum 4:95-150, 1974.
4. Woessner JF Jr. Mammalian collagenase. Clin Orthop 96:310-326, 1973.
5. Harris ED Jr, Krane SM. Collagenases. N Engl J Med 291:557-563, 1974.

OSTEOARTHRITIS

DAVID S. HOWELL, M.D.

DEFINITION AND INCIDENCE

Osteoarthritis (OA) or degenerative joint disease involves most commonly the knees, hips, bunion joints, proximal and distal interphalangeal joints of hands and feet, and first carpometacarpal joints (Fig. 1), as well as cervical, thoracic, and lumbosacral spine (Figs. 2 and 3). Most disabling lesions occur in the weight-bearing joints (1). When there is no known etiology, the term primary osteoarthritis is used.

Secondary osteoarthritis describes a clinical syndrome indistinguishable from the primary type except for related causative factors in initiating the local joint damage. The term has been used for osteoarthritis that follows fractures, severe sprains, chronic local infections, well-defined heritable diseases, and biomechanical derangement of articular function, as well as metabolic disorders such as ochronosis and chondrocalcinosis. Also, RA and its variants in an advanced stage often are accompanied by the joint changes of secondary osteoarthritis, i.e., "mixed arthritis." The estimated prevalence of OA in the United States assessed from x-rays of hands and feet during a health survey conducted from 1960 to 1962 was 40.5 million. By age 75, 85% of a population sampled in another survey were affected and 25% had moderate to severe disease. Sex incidence is equal. A form with clear hereditary features is the osteoarthritis of Kellgren. This involves a polyarthritis with distal and proximal interphalangeal joint involvement and strong hereditary factors.

PATHOLOGY AND PHYSIOLOGY

The disease is relatively noninflammatory (2) and, by definition, progressive. It is characterized by deterioration of the articular cartilage

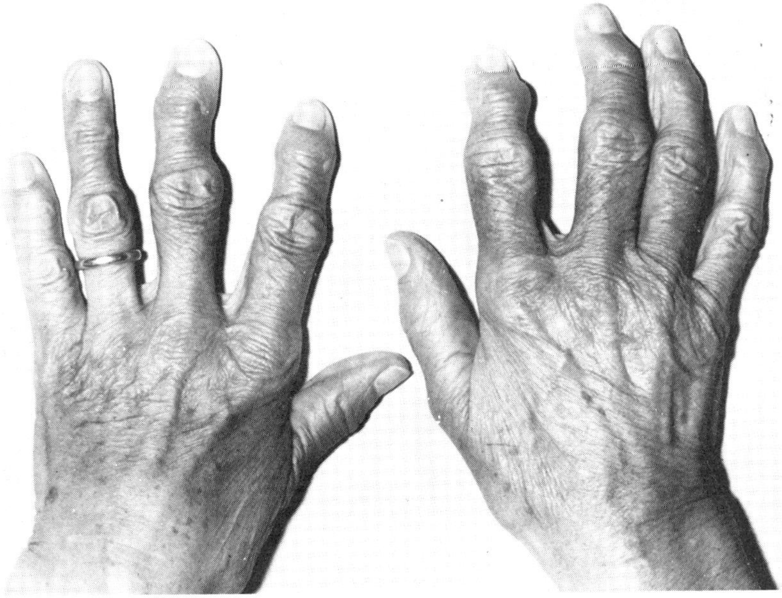

FIGURE 1
Well-developed changes of the hand in osteoarthritis.

FIGURE 2
Bridging of vertebrae with compression of bodies.

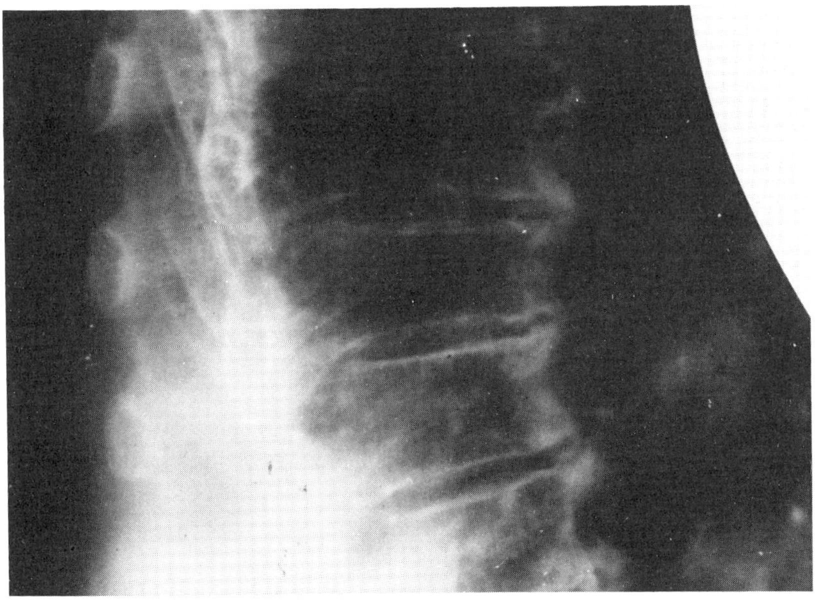

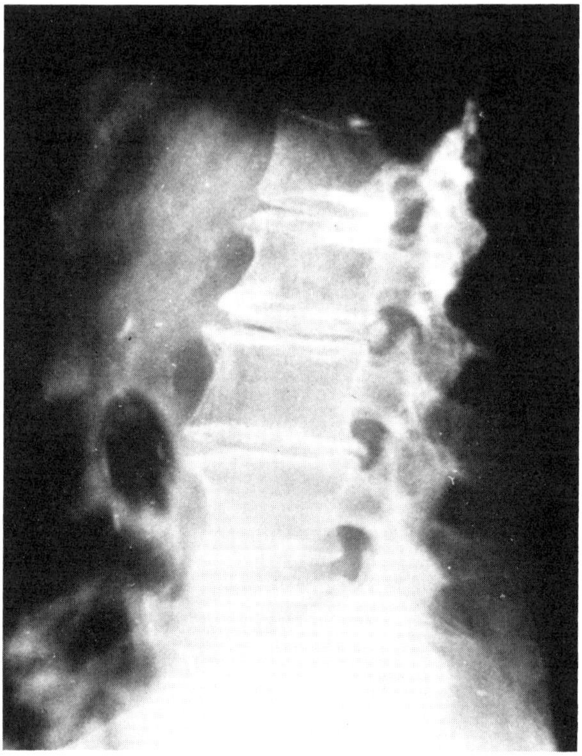

FIGURE 3
Extensive spur formation in bodies of vertebrae and narrowing of intervertebral disc space.

as well as formation of new bone in subchondral areas and rims of bone at the joint margins.

Articular cartilage is specialized connective tissue, normally made up of a small number of chondrocytes, lodged in an abundant extracellular matrix composed of collagen, proteoglycans, and glycoproteins. Cartilage cells must receive nutrients to support cellular and metabolic activities and discharge waste products of metabolism. In growing human beings, the sources of nutrition come from both the subchondral epiphyseal island and from synovial fluid. With disappearance of the growth cartilage in the epiphyseal plate, there is concurrent disappearance of the growth cartilage portion of the articular organ. The deep radial zone becomes calcified and separated from the uncalcified cartilage by a deeply staining line, the tidemark (2). Only a small amount, if any, of nutrition is supplied by the bone marrow after this stage of development. Thereafter, all nutrition is derived from the synovial fluid. Histologic studies indicate that cartilage is best preserved when subjected to intermittent compressive contact, such as in ordinary weight-bearing exercise. Atrophy of cartilage occurs during prolonged casting of patients. On the other hand, severe compressive contact, as in trauma, injures the cartilage.

Human and most animal models of OA appear similar, due to the limited number of histologic responses to noxious stimuli that the tissue can undergo. At first, there are yellow, opaque, or softened areas with roughening of the surface of the cartilage. The cracks spread along the plane of collagen fibers of the matrix, whose fibers are organized roughly into arcades. Minute fragments of cartilage break off into the synovial fluid, become phagocytized, and provoke a secondary acute or low grade chronic synovitis. Subchondral bone remodels with increased density, and a polished eburnated appearance occurs. Spurs of new bone called osteophytes grow at joint margins as well as at ligamentous and tendon attachment sites. Osteophytes may break off into the joint cavity and produce joint mice.

Normal cartilage histologically can stain strongly with saffranin O, a cationic dye that binds to sulfated proteoglycans. These proteoglycans comprise about 10–15% of the dry weight of the cartilage. They stain deep red. The rest of the cartilage depleted of the polysaccharides stains green. The collagen fibers are obscured by proteoglycans normally. Applying these stains to osteoarthritic cartilage, one recognizes an initial loss of staining reaction in the early osteoarthritic site. Cells degenerate and disappear in the upper layers of the cartilage, whereas nests of cells divide forming "brood capsules" (1).

Biochemical studies (3) indicate that in the normal adult there is chiefly an equal mixture of chondroitin-6-sulfate and keratan sulfate as the predominant glycosaminoglycans present. In some of the areas that appear stimulated to growth around the ulcerated cartilage and in the margins of the joints, there is evidence of altered concentrations of chondroitin-4-sulfate, chondroitin-6-sulfate, and keratan sulfate (4). Collagen does not appear to be broken down significantly in the early stages of OA. Concurrent with altered size of proteoglycans, increased activity of cathepsin D is registered in early osteoarthritic lesions. This enzyme, localized in the lysosomes, probably contributes in the last stages of breakdown of proteoglycans (5). This degradation is a feature accelerated in some osteoarthritic tissues together with compensatory increased proteoglycan synthesis (3). New drugs for this disease are sought that would either block the degradative enzymes or stimulate further adequate repair (5).

Mechanically, the osteoarthritic cartilage becomes less elastic, possibly due to subchondral bone thickening at an earlier stage than assumed previously (4). Loss of cartilage volume may lead to severe joint incongruity and joint instability, greatly accelerating the rate of cartilage breakdown. Ligaments become loosened in the process (4).

THEORIES ON PATHOGENESIS

The major current theories on pathogenesis are discussed in detail elsewhere (1,2,4–6). One theory concerns disposing microtrauma through the years, causing increased wear and tear, particularly at weight-bearing sites in cartilage. These sites include the commonly involved distal interphalangeal joints that receive considerable shocks in daily living. Theoretically, tissue surface breaks may appear that allow enzymes in the synovial fluid to initiate partial cartilage matrix degradation. In addition, the trauma probably injures the cells near the surface per se.

Neutral proteases are released throughout the matrix. The proteases break down the proteoglycans to smaller fragments that then diffuse through the matrix back to the cells, where the final degradation occurs in phagolysosomes by cathepsin D and perhaps other cathepsins; the latter enzymes work in a much more acid environment. This breakdown appears to turn on a cellular system of repair with synthesis of new glycoproteins and proteoglycans to restore those lost by degradation. This repair process is inadequate, however, and the inadequate matrix with poor mechanical properties becomes further degraded. The products of degradation are believed to stimulate in some manner the marginal and local bone cells to remodel and progenitor cells to differentiate into cells capable of influencing new bone formation. New fibrocartilage forms around the rims of the joints over the spurs. Some new fibrocartilage may also form after bone becomes denuded of cartilage and new bone marrow grows up into the ulcerated lesion.

A second theory involves the belief that microtrauma stiffens subcondral bone, leading to mechanical injury of the joints.

A third theory implicates failure of nutrition when joints become more congruous as the slight but important remodeling of aging occurs.

Finally, formation of ridges and angulations of joint contact in the hip and knee may have an important role in many cases of OA, findings which are believed to be developmental in nature.

CLINICAL FINDINGS

Joints become squared, firm, and tender. Usually there are few objective findings, so that evaluation of new agents or drugs are difficult. Synovial effusions in the knee and hip offer little of diagnostic value on aspiration. During acute attacks there will be warmth and redness, particularly in the hands over the distal interphalangeal joints (Heberden's nodes) or the proximal interphalangeal joints (Bouchard's nodes). The knee may also be mildly inflamed.

MANAGEMENT

Primary OA and other rheumatic disorders show greatly magnified symptoms. Possibly, the inflammatory components are worsened by the presence of chronic anxiety. Therefore, it is important to reassure the patient that he is not afflicted with a severe crippling disorder. This reassurance should follow a thorough internal and medical rheumatologic workup.

The prognosis is governed by the extent of involvement of weight-bearing sites. Usually, the hips are most difficult to treat by medical means and are least responsive to therapeutic agents. Prognosis is also governed in secondary osteoarthritis by the disease to which the condition is secondary.

MEDICAL MEASURES

Medical measures include partial relief of weight-bearing joint pain, usually accompanying weight loss. In the hips, effective pressures develop three times that of the actual weight of the body above the hips due to local biomechanical factors. Rest is important, along with formal stretching, postural exercise, and isometric tension exercises to improve the strength of muscles, and splinting of joints that have become lax. Overactivity of painful joints should be discouraged (7).

Drugs such as salicylates should initially be used: Tylenol, 0.6 to 0.9 g q.i.d., or Ecotrin, 3.6 to 4.8 g q.i.d. If these are ineffective, Darvon, 65 mg, 3 to 4 capsules per day, should be tried. Alternatively, Motrin,[1] 400 mg, 4 to 8 tablets per day may be used, or indomethacin, 25 mg t.i.d., may also be given along with antacids to protect against frequent gastrointestinal disturbances. If these agents are ineffective, phenylbutazone, 100 mg t.i.d. or q.i.d. with blood counts at 1, 2, and 4 weeks for the detection of possible bone marrow depression or aplastic anemia, should be tried. Phenylbutazone should not be used in the presence of allergic states, hypertension, or heart failure. Finally, if these measures fail, local corticosteroid injections, analgesics, and physical therapy, and even codeine or Percodan, may be required.

Local corticosteroid injections are indicated in the presence of inflammation and failure of response to aforementioned programs (7). Five or 6 injections over 4- to 6-week intervals in any single joint per 6- to 12-month period should be the limit, due to predictable unfavorable effects of the drug. Although corticosteroids stabilize lysosomes and may block a potential pathway of degradation involving hydrolytic enzymes in the chondrocytes, these agents hinder repair of the cartilage. Cystic degeneration and disintegration of the cartilage have been reported with overusage. Corticosteroids should not be used at sites near pustules, since septic arthritis may follow injection. Patients should be alerted that mild increased joint aching will occur at the injection site after the anesthetic has worn off. If severe pain occurs, such a crystal reaction will respond to phenylbutazone, ice packs, and analgesics.

Care taken in local corticosteroid injections, using fine needles and Xylocaine, produces better results than indicated by the sketchily described methods in most textbooks.

PHYSICAL THERAPY

Moist heat applied to painful Heberden's nodes for 20 min daily is effective. Infrared radiation heating, shortwave diathermy, ultrasound, and hot wet packs are frequently used in peripheral joints

---

[1]Motrin and other nonsteroidal agents such as Naprosyn, Tolectin, and Nalfon in equivalent dosages are usually preferable (depending on individual patient response in 7-10 day trials) to Butazolidin, in terms of potential toxicity.

as well as the back. Isometric exercises should be added to the program as pain relief occurs. Therapeutic swimming, 20 to 30 min daily, is an important asset. Gloves and Band-Aids to protect joints repeatedly microtraumatized are useful and simple measures often neglected. Metatarsal bars placed on oxfords or use of arch supports are recommended for painful feet with metatarsal prolapse. First carpometacarpal joints are aided with wrist supports after periarticular corticosteroid shots and light slings. Knee cages or elastic supports with hinged metal reinforcements are strongly recommended for painful knees. Canes, crutches, and walkers are used in more advanced cases (8).

SURGICAL INTERVENTION

Intractable pain, especially night pain, and extensive cartilage destruction with joint instability are indications for consulting the orthopedic surgeon (9). There is extensive use of new total hip replacement procedures revolutionized by plastic embedding of prostheses in bone. Otherwise, osteotomy of the hip or knee, or insertion of partial prosthetic devices in the knee are indicated, although total knee replacement may be necessary in advanced cases. Swollen boggy knees in which there is evidence of loose bodies by x-ray may be subjected to synovectomy and debridgement. Ligamentous repair and tightening at the knee is particularly helpful.

REFERENCES

1. Sokoloff L. The Biology of Degenerative Joint Disease. Chicago: University of Chicago Press, 1969.
2. Sokoloff L, Malemud CJ, Srivastava VML, Morgan WD. In vitro culture of articular chondrocytes. Fed Proc 32:1499–1502, 1973.
3. Mankin HJ, Dorman H, Lippiello L, et al. Biochemical and metabolic abnormalities in articular cartilage from osteoarthritic human hips: II. Correlation of morphology with biochemical and metabolic data. J Bone Joint Surg 53:523–537, 1971.
4. Howell DS, Sapolsky AI, Pita JC, et al. The pathogenesis of osteoarthritis. Semin Arthritis Rheum 5:365–383, 1976.
5. Howell DS. Degradative enzymes in osteoarthritic human articular cartilage. Pemberton Lecture. Arthritis Rheum 18:167–177, 1975.
6. Bollet AJ. An essay on the biology of osteoarthritis. Arthritis Rheum 12:152–163, 1969.

7. Howell DS, Altman RD, Brown HE Jr, et al. A comprehensive regimen for osteoarthritis. Med Clin North Am 55:457–469, 1971.
8. Marmor L. Surgery of osteoarthritis. Semin Arthritis Rheum 2:117–156, 1972.
9. Simon WH. The Human Joint in Health and Disease. Philadelphia: University of Pennsylvania Press, 1978.

LOW BACKACHE

DAVID S. HOWELL, M.D.

In a recent local hospital survey, concluding diagnoses of cause of low back pain were roughly 60% osteogenic or fibrogenic, 15% viscerogenic, 21% psychogenic and idiopathic, and 4% neurologic and vascular. An often difficult medical judgment in practice is to decide whether a low backache represents only a minor idiopathic derangement or, in contrast, whether important organic factors are causal.

Definitive minor psychogenic or idiopathic derangements can be handled on an outpatient basis, whereas suspicion of serious internal medical causes or recalcitrant disc syndromes usually warrant hospitalization. The usual sequence with such a case is to obtain a careful internal and rheumatologic workup as well as orthopedic and neurologic evaluation.

The most common cause of osteogenic backache is of structural nature, including mostly degenerative disorders, some posttraumatic (sprain syndromes), and a few developmental ones. The next most common cause includes the rheumatoid variants, followed by metabolic disorders, infections, and neoplasms. The most common form of the degenerative low back lesion is spondylosis, an all-inclusive term that describes degeneration of the intervertebral disc and annulus fibrosis with pressure of one or both structures on the spinal cord or nerve rootlets, foraminal spurs with pressure on nerve rootlets, disc collapse and traction on nerve rootlets, subacute synovitis of the facets and related ligaments and tendons, as well as nerve entrapment by paraspinal ligaments and tendons. Radiologic study may bring out additional or separate developmental abnormalities such as spondylolisthesis, absent or abnormal facets, arches, and sacralization or lumbarization at L5-S1 levels (1).

The diagnosis of spondylosis is made by suitable exclusion of other diseases, registration of nerve deficits in lower limbs by combinations of careful neurologic examinations (often with electromyography), response to 3 weeks of bedrest, and, finally, axial tomography or myelography to show spinal stenosis. Present as an accompaniment of minor low back derangement but also often associated with spondylosis are tense paravertebral muscles and variable additional components such as localized fibromyositis, herniated fat pads, trochanteric and gluteal bursitis, as well as trigger points. These features often clear up spontaneously on bedrest, physiotherapy, and other symptomatic treatment.

Rheumatoid variants include ankylosing spondylitis and spondylitis associated with psoriasis, Reiter's syndrome, and ulcerative colitis. Characteristic radiologic changes can be observed in the sacroiliac joints and apophyseal rotary joints of the spine.

Metabolic bone disease is dependent on radiologic findings (e.g., those of Paget's disease, osteoporosis with compression fracture, and osteomalacia). Neoplasms such as multiple myeloma; metastatic tumors to bone, particularly from the kidney, thyroid, or breast; sarcoma; and osteoid osteoma must be considered. Vertebral infections are most uncommon but should not be disregarded. These include acute *E. coli* infection, staphylococcus infection with vertebral involvement or chronic typhoid fever, and *Brucella* disease. Nonpyogenic granuloma, tuberculosis, and actinomycosis should also be sought.

Viscerogenic causes of low backache should be considered early. Genitourinary tract lesions are common, including nephrolithiasis, infection, and nephroptosis. In female pelvic viscera, endometriosis, chronic cervicitis, and retroverted uterus are common. Finally, retropharyngeal sacromas, hiatus hernia, duodenal ulcer, and pancreatitis must be considered as causes of referred backache.

Primary psychogenic disorders such as conversion hysteria or psychogenic regional pain, or secondary ones including anxiety states, depression, "tension rheumatism," personality defects, and compensation neurosis, may be implicated.

Dissecting or localized aneurysms, cord tumor, vascular thrombosis, etc. comprise minor but important causes of backache as it presents to the internist.

In general, serious disease, whether due to vertebral compression, metabolic bone disease, discogenic pressure, or tumor, results in a neurologic deficit with respect to the innervation of the lower extremities and bladder. This will appear as pain referred from the spine to various dermatomes with a prevalence of sciatica in discogenic L5-S1 disease and loss of knee or ankle jerks, as well as loss of flexion at the ankle and muscle atrophy (2). Neurogenic bladder dysfunction may occur and should be investigated by cystometrograms if there are symptoms of urinary retention. After visceral and vascular causes are excluded, in the absence of true neurologic deficits, intractable disc disease or spinal stenosis may be present (3).

Rest; modalities of physical therapy such as hot packs, ultrasound, massage, and, in some cases, use of traction; muscle relaxants; mild sedation; and analgesics during a 7–10 day period in bed should be tried. A poor response to this management prompts consideration of first, noninvasive diagnostic procedures (e.g., high resolution computerized axial tomography); second, invasive diagnostic procedures (e.g., paravertebral venogram, discogram, and myelography). Details of such management are described elsewhere (1–3).

REFERENCES

1. Coventry MD. Anatomy of the intervertebral disc. Clin Orthop 67:9–15, 1969.
2. Armstrong JR. Lumbar Disc Lesions. 3rd ed. Baltimore: Williams & Wilkins, 1965.
3. Kirkaldy-Willis WH, McIvor GWD. Spinal stenosis. Symposium. Clin Orthop 115:2–3, 1976.
4. Brown MD. Low back strain and rupture of the intervertebral disk: treatment of painful back syndromes. In: Practice of Surgery. Vol. 2, Chapter 14. New York: Harper & Row, 1977.

BURSITIS, TENDONITIS, AND FIBROSITIS

WILBUR J. BLECHMAN, M.D.

Bursae are connective tissue-lined sacs that secrete a lubricating fluid resembling synovial fluid and prevent friction between moving parts of connective tissue, such as muscles and tendons. Trauma is the most common cause of bursitis. Frequently this occurs as repetitive microtrauma or excessive friction and has a relationship to occupation or hobbies. The end result is an inflamed bursa with edema and pain, at times disabling. Inflammatory forms of arthritis (RA, Reiter's syndrome, ankylosing spondylitis, gout, etc.) are other common causes, most often involving the olecranon or Achilles area. Infection is a less frequent cause but must always be considered.

BURSITIS

Frequent sites of bursitis include:

1. *Subdeltoid.* The usual shoulder bursitis. This is generally acute and often is due to rupture of an adjacent calcific deposit on an inflamed tendon. There may or may not be objective signs of inflammation, but the patient does not usually allow either active or passive motion of the arm. Exquisite local tenderness is present.
2. *Olecranon.* Actual pain may be mild to moderate or even absent. Often it is the obvious swelling that sends the patient to the doctor. Nodules or tophi may be present when RA or gout is the underlying disorder.
3. *Ischial.* Weaver's bottom. Buttock pain and nerve root-like pain may predominate, mimicking a radiculitis; however, local tenderness is apparent and is best detected with the patient lying on the side with hips flexed.

4. *Trochanteric.* This is common and often misdiagnosed as a hip arthritis or a radiculitis. It is more common in women and in the elderly or obese. Subtle changes in gait (at times even from changing shoes) may play a causative role.
5. *Calcaneal.* Though trauma is the most common cause, this is a frequently involved site in RA and the B-27 positive group of arthropathies.
6. *Anserine.* Often associated with coincidental osteoarthritis of the knee, this is another common, but frequently overlooked, source of pain. Persistent pain after treatment of knee osteoarthritis may be due to bursal involvement. Gait and posture abnormalities play a causative or contributory role and must be treated for optimal results.

TENDONITIS (OR TENDINITIS)

Tendons and their sheathes also provide more than their share of problems. Trauma is the leading etiological agent, but the same diseases that affect bursae can also involve tendons and tendon sheaths. Local tenderness and pain on motion occur. Swelling and crepitus may be noted. Some common forms include:

1. *Bicipital tendonitis.* May coexist with rotator cuff disease and may progress to an adhesive capsulitis. Rolling the bicipital tendon under the fingertips in the bicipital groove at the anterior aspect of the humeral head usually discloses marked tenderness.
2. *Tennis elbow.* Considered to be a tendonitis of the origin of the extensor tendons at the lateral epicondyle of the humerus. Any activity associated with repetitive wrist extension or pronation-supination may be causative.
3. *Carpal tunnel syndrome.* Frequently overlooked as a cause of hand discomfort. The patient complains of pain in the hand, but when pressed for specifics the patient describes a painful numbness and tingling of the first three or four fingers, worse at night and with activity. Pain may radiate into the forearm or even to the shoulder. Tinel's and/or Phalen's signs are frequently, but not invariably, present.
4. *DeQuervain's disease.* Due to a stenosing tenosynovitis, it leads to complaints of pain in the region of the radial styloid. Patients have a weak grip plus a positive Finkelstein sign.

5. *Trigger fingers.* Result from nodular enlargement of the flexor tendons.

TREATMENT

Appropriate rest and exercise patterns plus the use of local corticosteroids, nonsteroidal antiinflammatory drugs, and physical therapy measures are usually helpful, singly or in combination, in both tendon and bursa disorders. At times, however, surgery may be necessary, especially if stenosing tenosynovitis or nerve entrapment is present. If inflammation is secondary to underlying disease, treatment must also be directed to that condition.

FIBROSITIS

Fibrositis describes a symptom complex manifested by aching, stiffness, soreness, pain, and tenderness involving primarily the musculoskeletal soft tissues of neck, shoulders, back, hips, and proximal extremities. Symptoms are frequently aggravated by emotional and physical stress, fatigue, weather changes, cold, and activity. Patients claim poor sleeping habits and feel worse on arising. An increase in tenderness of specific muscle areas and a coincident disturbance in non-REM sleep has been confirmed. Sleep disturbance and exaggerated tenderness at anatomically reproducible locations indicate the presence of a definable syndrome.

Other than tenderness and a frequent finding of anxiety, with or without depression, physical examination may be remarkable in its normality. Blood studies will be normal unless coexistent disease is present. X-ray and muscle biopsy are not helpful.

Therapy is frequently unsatisfactory. The physician must consider and utilize diverse forms of treatment for best results. The response of each patient must be evaluated individually. Treatment forms may include nonsteroidal antiinflammatory drugs, nonnarcotic analgesics, ethyl chloride spray, physical therapy modalities, and local steroid-lidocaine injections. In some instances relief has been reported following use of transcutaneous electrical stimulation, acupuncture, and biofeedback. Use of chlorpromazine for insomnia has also been helpful in reducing the overall pain.

CHONDROCALCINOSIS

DAVID S. HOWELL, M.D.

Chondrocalcinosis is a chronic form of arthritis with recurrent acute attacks that resemble, in many respects, those of uric acid gouty arthritis. The term pseudogout should be confined to the description of the acute inflammatory attack and should be accompanied by identifiable calcium pyrophosphate crystals in the synovial fluid both within leukocytes and free floating. Chondrocalcinosis is also identified by histologic stains for calcium salt in the articular cartilage, by dense bands in the cartilage running parallel with the subchondral bone plate seen by x-ray (Fig. 1), and, most conclusively, by x-ray diffraction study of mineral crystals isolated from diseased joints (1). Heritable forms have been found in family aggregations in the Chiloe Islands off Chile and in Czechoslovakia (2,3).

The form seen in the United States usually develops over age 50 years with a preponderance of males. At least 66% of the patients have osteoarthritis indistinguishable from that of the primary osteoarthritis. However, many of these patients have the additional distinctive feature of chondrocalcinotic lesions sometimes found in carpal and metacarpal bones, sites rarely afflicted with typical osteoarthritis (3). Thus, for the majority of patients, the principal pathologic problem is that of the accompanying OA. In a minority there is considerable disablement from recurrent acute episodes of inflammatory pseudogout, most commonly in the knees.

Chondrocalcinosis and pseudogout are also seen in diseases where there are metabolic errors that might contribute to the deposition of calcium pyrophosphate. These are hemochromatosis, hyperparathyroidism, Wilson's disease, ochronosis, diabetes mellitus, and uric acid gouty arthritis.

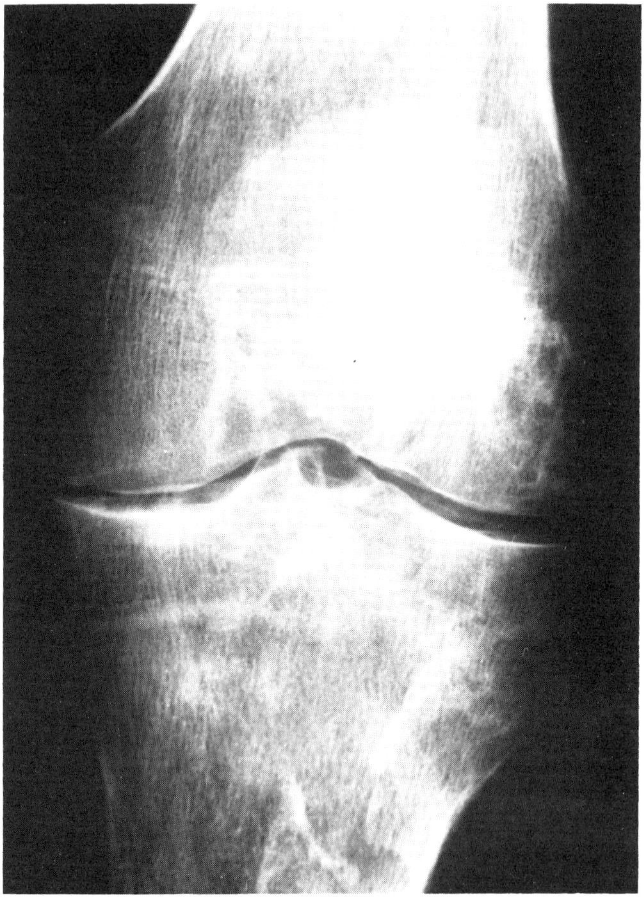

FIGURE 1
Deposits of calcium in lateral meniscus.

The cause of crystal deposition in chondrocalcinosis is unknown. Serum alkaline phosphatase and urinary pyrophosphate excretion are normal. Elevated synovial fluid pyrophosphate concentrations have been reported in comparison to normal synovial fluid (4). It has been postulated that the final common defect may be a deficiency or inhibition of cartilage pyrophosphates (5).

Treatment usually consists of a nonsteroidal antiinflammatory agent such as indomethacin, 200 mg per day for 3 days. Substitution of other antiinflammatory agents may be advisable in both the acute attack and interval treatment. Joint aspiration per se may give relief during acute attacks with an effusion.

REFERENCES

1. McCarty DJ Jr, Hogan JM, Gatter RA, Grossman M. Studies on pathological calcifications in human cartilage: I. Prevalence and types of crystal deposits in the menisci of two hundred fifteen cadavera. J Bone Joint Surg 48A:309-325, 1966.
2. Zitnan D, Sitaj S. Chondrocalcinosis articularis, Section I: Clinical and radiological study. Ann Rheum Dis 22:142-152, 1963.
3. McCarty DJ Jr, ed. Chondrocalcinosis and pseudogout. Symposium. Arthritis Rheum 19:No. 3 suppl. 275-285, 1976.
4. Altman RD, Muniz O, Pita JC, Howell DS. Articular chondrocalcinosis microanalysis of pyrophosphate (PPi) in synovial fluid and plasma. Arthritis Rheum 16:171-178, 1973.
5. Howell DS, Muniz O, Pita JC, Enis JE. Extrusion of pyrophosphate into extracellular media by osteoarthritic cartilage incubates. J Clin Invest 56:1473-1480, 1975.

HEMOCHROMATOSIS

ROY D. ALTMAN, M.D.

Hemochromatosis is a chronic disease characterized by excess iron deposition with associated fibrosis in many tissues with eventual functional impairment of several organs (e.g., liver, pancreas) in untreated patients. Frequently encountered clinical manifestations include hepatomegaly and cirrhosis, skin pigmentation, diabetes mellitus, other endocrine dysfunctions, and heart failure associated with a familial pattern. Arthropathy occurs in 20% of patients. There is elevation of serum iron concentration and saturation of plasma iron-binding protein transferrin.

SECONDARY DEGENERATIVE ARTHROPATHY

An arthropathy associated with hemochromatosis was first described by Schumacher and occurs in 20 to 50% of patients with hemochromatosis (1). Average age of onset is in the sixth decade, with a range of 26 to 70 years of age. Onset of arthropathy is usually simultaneous with the onset of other symptoms of the disease. However, the joint symptoms may precede other characteristics of increased iron stores (2) and may be confused with rheumatoid arthritis. Joint symptoms may also occur late in the course of the disease, even when treated.

Hands, knees, and hips are most frequently involved. Characteristic hand findings are a firm, only mildly tender, enlargement of metacarpophalangeal (MCP), proximal (PIP), and distal interphalangeal (DIP) joints. As in rheumatoid arthritis, the second and third MCP joints are most often affected. Hand x-rays often also show the following characteristic involvement of MCP, PIP, and DIP joints:

narrowing of the joint space, cystlike erosions, joint space irregularity, subchondral sclerosis, and moderate bony proliferation (3).

Synovial fluid is noninflammatory with low leukocyte counts and predominantly mononuclear cells, good viscosity, and pale yellow color. Occasional mononuclear cells in the synovium fluid can be shown to contain iron by Prussian blue stain (4). Biopsy of synovial tissue shows a striking deposition of iron predominantly in the synovial lining cells. Because of synovial hemosiderin deposition in other diseases, diagnosis may warrant histologic study of a liver biopsy.

SECONDARY CHONDROCALCINOSIS

Chondrocalcinosis occurs in up to 30% of patients with hemochromatosis and is usually associated with degenerative arthropathy (5). It can also be an isolated joint finding. Calcification is more commonly detected in menisci and articular cartilages at the knee, but may also be seen at the wrists, fingers, elbows, shoulders, hips, ankles, toes, symphysis pubis, intervertebral discs, and in the soft tissue of the heels or elsewhere. An acute or chronic arthritis with synovial fluid crystals identified as calcium pyrophosphate can occur, pointing to a diagnosis of pseudogout. The synovial effusion is usually inflammatory during such episodes. The crystal deposits in the cartilage are calcium. Iron staining of cartilage has also been seen, but this is only in chondrocytes and at the line of ossification (6).

OSTEOPENIA

Diffuse demineralization of bone occurs in 25 to 50% of patients, but its relationship to the hemochromatosis is unclear. Diffuse osteopenia of the hands is most common.

Therapy of the arthropathy of hemochromatosis is largely symptomatic, directed at the specific problems.

REFERENCES

1. Schumacher HR Jr. Hemochromatosis and arthritis. Arthritis Rheum 7:41-50, 1964.
2. M'Seffar A, Fornasier VL, Fox IH. Arthropathy as the major clinical indicator of occult iron storage disease. JAMA 238:1825-1828, 1977.

3. Hirsch JH, Killien FC, Troupin RH. The arthropathy of hemochromatosis. Radiology 188:591-596, 1976.
4. Schumacher HR Jr. Ultrastructural characteristics of the synovial membrane in idiopathic haemochromatosis. Ann Rheum Dis 31:465-473, 1972.
5. Hamilton EBD. Diseases associated with CPPD deposition disease. Arthritis Rheum 19:353-357, 1976.
6. Brighton CT, Bidley EC, Smolensky BI. Iron induced arthritis in immature rabbits. Arthritis Rheum 13:849-857, 1970.

OCHRONOSIS

NORMAN L. GOTTLIEB, M.D.

Ochronosis is a rare hereditary disorder characterized by alkaptonuria (homogentisic acid in the urine that turns brownish-black when oxidized) and connective tissue pigmentation involving most prominently the cartilage of the ear, skin, sclera, and hyaline articular cartilage (1). Alkaptonuria denotes the affinity of homogentisic acid in alkaline solution for oxygen, resulting in polymerization of homogentisic acid, which is responsible for the pigmentary change. Alkaptonuria is asymptomatic, but pigment deposition in connective tissues usually results in clinical signs and symptoms (2).

ETIOLOGY

The biochemical defect responsible for alkaptonuria and ochronosis is the absence of homogentisic acid oxidase in the metabolic pathway of the aromatic amino acid tyrosine. This enzyme converts homogentisic acid to maleylacetoacetic acid in the liver. Current evidence suggests that ochronosis is transmitted by a single recessive autosomal gene resulting from consanguineous marriages, accounting for its occurrence in successive generations of affected families.

CLINICAL FINDINGS

The major clinical manifestations of ochronosis include pigmentary changes, spondylosis, and peripheral arthropathy; less frequently, cardiovascular and prostatic abnormalities are seen (3). Most patients with alkaptonuria who survive the fourth decade develop ochronosis. The cartilage of the ear becomes irregularly thickened, inflexible, and slate blue. The outer rim of the tympanic membrane may appear grayish-black and the cerumen black. Some patients suffer from impaired hearing. Scleral pigmentation usually is localized between the corneal limbus and the inner or outer canthi. Skin pigmentation occurs most commonly over the malar region, nose, axilla, and groin.

Spondylosis develops in most ochronotic patients by age 30; symptoms include low back pain and stiffness. As with Marie-Strümpell's

FIGURE 1

Black pigment is deposited in all the intervertebral discs of the lumbar spine, which are decreased in volume and irregularly outlined, in a patient with ochronosis. Bony ankylosis at the margins of some discs, and one focus of intervertebral ossification, is shown.

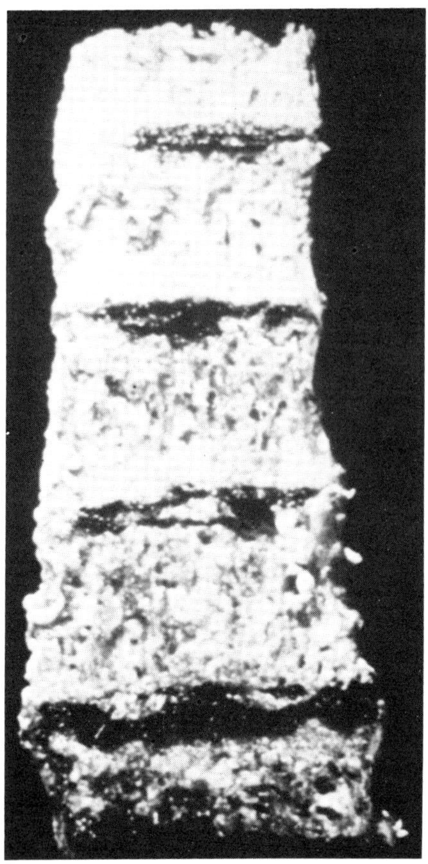

disease, lumbar involvement occurs initially, progressively involving the dorsal and finally the cervical spine. Loss of lumbar lordosis, spinal rigidity, and kyphosis may occur; occasionally roentgenographic findings are marked while symptoms are minimal. Calcification or ossification of the intravertebral discs is characteristic, at times associated with narrowing of intravertebral disc spaces and small osteophytes (Fig. 1). These findings are not specific for ochronosis. In contrast to Marie-Strümpell's disease, the sacroiliac and apophyseal joints are normal; a bamboo spine is not characteristic.

FIGURE 2

Synovial membrane from the knee of an ochronotic patient shows fragments of displaced pigmented articular cartilage, which have provoked a mild foreign body inflammatory reaction.

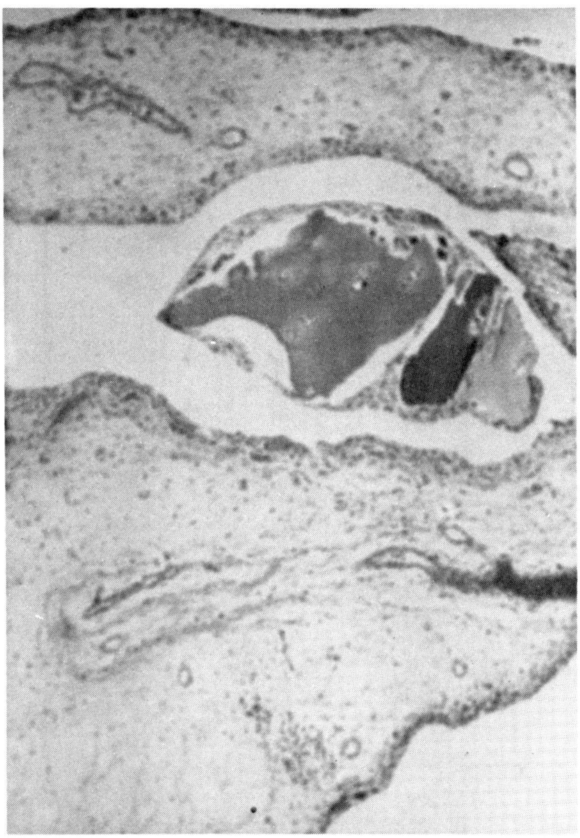

The peripheral arthropathy of ochronosis is degenerative, with pain, swelling, crepitation, and flexion contractures, which usually involve the knees, shoulders, and hips. Synovial fluid examination shows a clear, viscous, yellow fluid with a slight elevation in leukocyte count. Homogentisic acid may be demonstrated in the synovial fluid but in much lower concentrations than in urine. Synovial fluid usually does not darken on exposure to alkali, although some cells contain dark inclusions that may be phagocytosed ochronotic pigment: calcium pyrophosphate crystals may be seen (4). Cartilage degeneration and brittleness may be associated with fragmentation and pigmented shards in the synovium and osteochondral loose joint bodies (Fig. 2). Roentgenographic findings suggest primary osteoarthritis with joint space narrowing, osteophytosis, and juxtaarticular sclerosis; occasionally there is ossification of the paraarticular ligaments. The small joints of the hands and feet rarely are involved, in contrast to primary degenerative arthritis and some types of inflammatory arthritis. Recent evidence suggests that homogentisic acid inhibits the intracellular hydroxylation of lysine in collagen, which may be an important mechanism of cartilage deterioration (5).

PATHOLOGY

The pathologic lesions of ochronosis are secondary to the inter- or intracellular deposition of pigment, the exact composition of which is unknown. Some evidence suggests it is a polymer derived from homogentisic acid. Highly insoluble melaninlike granules may be found in the skin, subcutaneous tissues, cartilage, intervertebral discs, tracheal cartilage, and epithelial cells of the renal tubules, pancreas, arteries, and arterioles (Figs. 1 and 2).

TREATMENT

The treatment of ochronosis is primarily symptomatic; attempts to compensate for homogentisic acid oxidase deficiency have been unsuccessful. Diets low in phenylalanine and tryosine, reduced protein intake, and high doses of ascorbic acid have not been helpful. Similarly, systemic corticosteroids, radiation therapy, tyrosinase, and phenylbutazone are not beneficial. Analgesics, braces, limitation of joint use and abuse, weight reduction, and corrective orthopedic procedures may provide symptomatic relief.

REFERENCES

1. Schumacher HR, Holdsworth DE. Ochronotic arthropathy: I. Clinicpathologic studies. Semin Arthritis Rheum 6:207–246, 1977.
2. O'Brien WM, Bunim JJ. Biochemical, pathological, and clinical aspects of alkaptonuria, ochronosis, and ochronotic arthropathy: review of the world literature. Am J Med 34:813–838, 1963.
3. Steiger U, Lagier R. Combined anatomical and radiological study of the hip joint in alkaptonuric arthropathy. Ann Rheum Dis 31:369–373, 1972.
4. Reginato AJ, Schumacher HR, Martinez VA. Ochronotic arthropathy with calcium pyrophosphate crystal deposition. Arthritis Rheum 16:705–714, 1973.
5. Murray JC, Linberg KA, Pinnell SR. Inhibition of lysylhydroxylase by homogentisic acid: a proposed connective tissue defect in alkaptonuria. Clin Res 24:15A, 1976.

PAGET'S DISEASE

ROY D. ALTMAN, M.D.

In 1876, Sir James Paget presented a treatise entitled "On a form of chronic inflammation of bones (osteitis) deformans" (1). This malady, usually called "Paget's disease of bone" is a relatively common disorder with an average incidence of 149 per 100,000 hospitalized patients, or about 3% of a population over 40 years of age in Great Britain. Paget's disease is a chronic abnormality of the adult skeleton in which localized areas of hyperactive bone are replaced by a softened and enlarged osseous structure. Involved bones have a tendency to bowing, fracture, and, occasionally, malignant degeneration (Figs. 1–4). Although this disorder is common in its subclinical form, widespread, deforming, or disabling disease is uncommon. Many patients remain asymptomatic, but with more extensive involvement there is pain referable to the skull, axial skeleton, hips, and knees (2).

PATHOLOGY AND PATHOPHYSIOLOGY

Paget's disease is characterized by discrete pathologic lesions, often in multiple sites, with coarsely woven thickened lamellae and trabeculae with excessive osteoblastic and osteoclastic activity. There is considerable variation in the osteoclast size. The osteoclasts often contain several nuclei and inclusions suggesting an RNA virus. There is consequent extreme elevation of bone formation and resorption rates, which are reflected in high output of urinary hydroxyproline peptides, in elevated serum alkaline phosphatase, and in abnormal uptake of radionuclear technetium phosphate scanning agents of involved bones. Differences in overall mineral balance provide little information as to the extent of activity of disease. The commonest

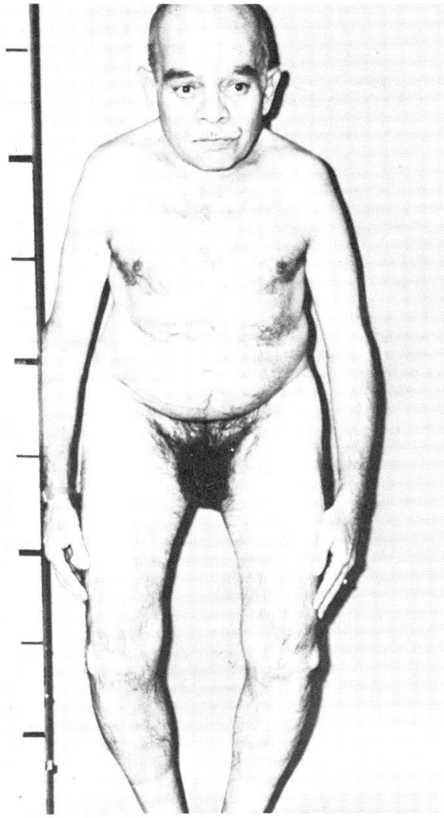

FIGURE 1

Paget's disease. Anterior view. Note the short stature, frontal bossing, simian posture, flared pelvis, and anterior and lateral bow to thighs and legs.

sites of predelection are pelvic and sacrum, femur, tibia, skull, lumbar and dorsal vertebrae, and clavicle. However, virtually any bone in the body may be diseased. There is a slight preponderance of lesions on the right side of the body.

Afflicted long bones may become structurally weakened with a tendency to deformity and fracture. Fracture of long bones may be complete or incomplete (microfractures, infractions). Compression fractures of vertebrae may also occur. Rapid bone replacement by the pagetic process may lead to bony enlargement that may induce a compression neuropathy. Paget's disease juxtaposited to an articula-

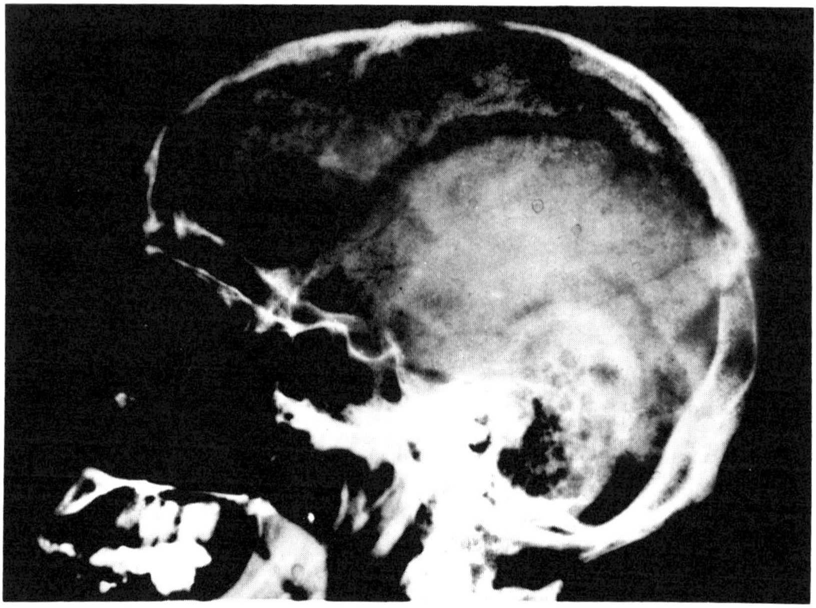

FIGURE 2
Skull x-ray osteoporosis circumscripta. Note linear area of temporal osteolytic Paget's disease.

tion may lead to degenerative joint disease. Extensive and active bone remodelling is associated with a local increased bony blood flow; a resultant high-output cardiac state with/without cardiac failure may develop. Sarcomatous degeneration occurs in less than 1% of patients, which is 40 times the frequency of a non-Paget's population. These tumors are usually osteogenic sarcomas encompassing varying histologic cell types.

CLINICAL FEATURES

The disease has a slight male predominance (1.5:1). In more than 80% of cases it is detected above the age of 50. It is almost exclusively in Caucasians and is particularly common in both Eastern and Western Europe. The etiology is unknown, but recent evidence suggests a viral infection. There is a familial tendency, but no genetic pattern has yet been defined.

Most often the disease is asymptomatic. Often the diagnosis is made by the incidental finding of an elevated serum alkaline phosphatase or

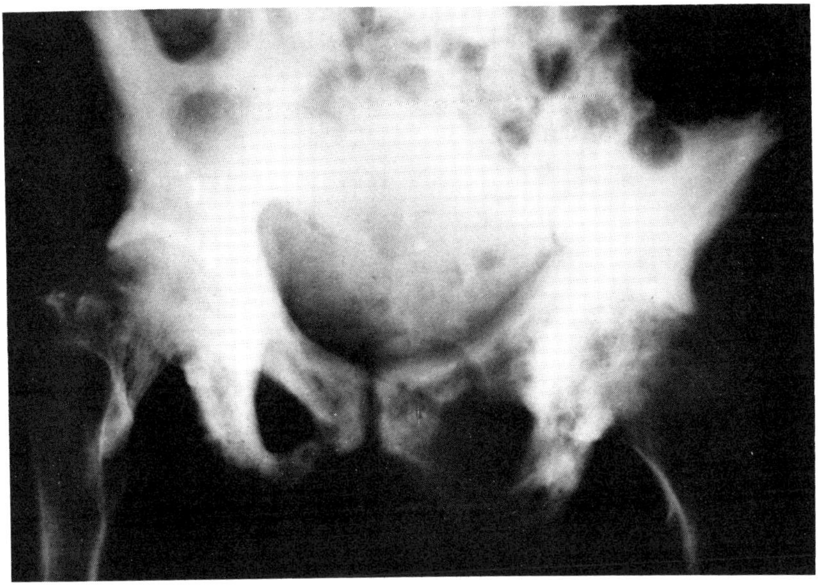

FIGURE 3

X-ray of pelvis. Note diffuse lytic, blastic, and fibrotic changes of Paget's disease of entire pelvis. There are coarse trabeculations and massive widening of the iliopectineal line.

by a roentgenogram for other purposes. The diagnosis may be made when the patient presents with a fracture through a pagetic site, the most common serious complication of the disease.

When symptoms occur, their onset is insidous. Clinical manifestations may often be realized only after 20–30 years (or more) of disease. They include general stiffness and fatigability, deformity, pain, headaches, dizziness, tinnitus, decreased auditory and/or visual acuity, increased skull size, excessive heat over a long bone or clavicle. Pain in Paget's bones is aching, deep, occasionally severe, and reminiscent of osteomalacic bone pain and may be accentuated at night. Often pain arises from compression neuropathy or associated secondary arthritis. In the presence of osteoarthritis, one must use caution in attributing pain to juxtaarticular Paget's disease.

Signs of the disease may be bitemporal skull enlargement with frontal "bossing," dilated scalp veins, nerve deafness, or otosclerosis in one or both ears with/without vestibular signs, angioid streaks of the optical fundus, a short kyphotic trunk with simian appearance and hob-

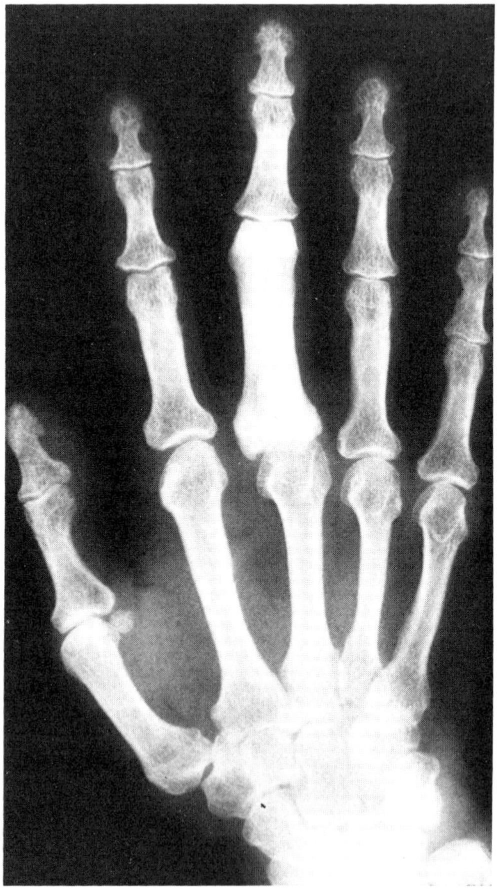

FIGURE 4

X-ray of hand. Note solitary third proximal phalanx involved with blastic pagetic changes. The bone is enlarged in vertical and horizontal planes.

bling gait, and anterolateral bow of the thigh or leg with warmth of periosteal tenderness. Intensity of symptoms and signs are highly variable.

The initial radiologic lesion is a radiolucent zone of bone resorption that follows the histologic pattern. This "lytic" zone is replaced by a coarse, heavy abnormal appearing trabecular pattern, frequently heavily calcified and accompanied by enlargement of the external contours of the bone. The bone scan is useful in delineating the extent of Paget's disease as the active pagetic sites accumulate intense amounts of nuclide, usually in excess of that usually accumulated by malignancy and to a more extensive area of bone than most malignancy.

DIAGNOSIS

Paget's disease should be readily distinguishable from other disorders in the advanced stages. Serum alkaline phosphatase should be elevated in active Paget's disease unless the disease is restricted. Serum and urine calcium determinations are normal unless immobilization has accelerated calcium absorption from bone. Paget's disease must be differentiated from metastatic prostatic carcinoma when serum acid phosphatase is elevated. Extreme elevation of serum acid phosphatase is uncommon in Paget's disease. Radioimmunoassay for prostatic acid phosphatase may be helpful. Only an occasional patient will need bone biopsy to differentiate Paget's disease from other bone disease, unless there is progressive severe pain and/or radiologic suggestion of primary or metastatic malignant disease. There is no current method that consistently differentiates serum alkaline phosphatase related to bone anabolism from other sources, e.g., liver. If the leucine aminopeptidase is elevated, hepatic origin of the alkaline phosphatase is suggested.

TREATMENT

Most often the disease is localized and asymptomatic and requires no treatment. Therapy is often aimed at the correction of a specific complication such as neural compression. When symptoms, such as pain, can be defined as bony (pagetic) in origin, suppressive therapy may be in order. Salicylates are effective analgesics, and nonsteroidal antiinflammatory agents may reduce pain of osteoarthritis. These therapies share a common property of suppressing some of the metabolic events by which bone cells remodel bone (particularly osteoclasts) and often influence mineral ion fluxes.

Calcitonin is a polypeptide hormone of ultimobranchial gland origin produced in human thyroid parafollicular cells. Although the precise physiologic role of the hormone in calcium homeostasis in human beings remains to be determined, numerous studies indicate important pharmacologic properties. Calcitonin produces a decrease in blood calcium levels. It has been used in several clinical studies to lower the serum calcium in hypercalcemic states. Several studies, both in vivo and in vitro, favor as primary, inhibitory action on bone resorption. Trials with parenteral administration of porcine calcitonin in generalized Paget's disease of bone have led to the conclusion that calcitonin is capable of producing a significant suppressive influence on the disease.

Beneficial clinical results have included reduction of bone pain, neurologic dysfunction, and congestive heart failure, as well as regression of bone lesions. Decreases in serum alkaline phosphatase, urinary hydroxyproline, and urinary calcium excretion have also been reported in long-term studies on the use of daily porcine calcitonin for periods up to 12 months, but initial therapeutic effects could not be sustained in a significant number of patients. Salmon calcitonin appears effective for 18 to 24 months. It was suggested that a limited effect was due either to secondary hyperparathyroidism induced by mild hypocalcemic effect of calcitonin or to neutralizing antibody formation or both. The most common side effect is an erythematous blush following administration of the drug. This often recedes with prolonged therapy or decreased dose and is rarely a cause for discontinuing the drug. Synthetic human calcitonin is not associated with tachyphylaxis or antibody formation.

Synthetic salmon calcitonin (Calcimar) is administered as 50–100 MRC subcutaneously at intervals ranging from daily to once weekly. Synthetic human calcitonin (Cibacalcin), available in Europe, is administered as 0.5–1 mg either daily or every other day.

Disodium etidronate, or EHDP (Didronel), is a compound related to pyrophosphate (6). It contains a molecular backbone of P–C–P (etidronate) instead of P–O–P (pyrophosphate) bonds of pyrophosphate. Development of this agent for therapeutic purposes is based on knowledge of pyrophosphate, an endogenous factor of theoretical regulatory importance in bone metabolism. Pyrophosphate, an anion formed as a ubiquitous end product of cell metabolism, circulates in small amounts in body fluids and is normally hydrolyzed by pyrophosphates. Pyrophosphate has been shown to inhibit both formation and dissolution of hydroxyapatite crystals in vitro.

A major action of pyrophosphate is considered to be the formation of a film on exposed mineral surfaces of bone under physiologic conditions with marked retardation of excretion or loss of mineral ions. Evidence has been obtained for an additional action of pyrophosphate, i.e., potent inhibition of conversion to hydroxyapatite crystals of noncrystalline (amorphous) calcium phosphate, considered to form initially in bone. Despite these effects of pyrophosphate in bone, exogenous administration of pyrophosphate was found to be of limited therapeutic value because of its rapid enzymatic destruction by endogenous pyrophosphatases. In contrast, the diphosphonates, which also form a film or chemisorb on the surface of bone minerals, are not hydrolyzed by pyrophosphatases. They maintain prolonged inhibitory activity of about the same type as that caused by pyrophosphate.

Recent evidence indicates that different diphosphonates may have additional modes of action. For example, there is some evidence that diphosphonates may exert a direct cellular effect on bone in vivo. Several investigators, including Altman and coworkers (5), found that disodium etidronate was effective in reducing pain, serum alkaline phosphatase, and urinary hydroxyproline in active Paget's disease. Prolonged benefit was noted after a single course of therapy in 33% of cases (6). Apparent side effects were limited to abdominal cramps. There did not appear to be any reduction in the incidence of fractures. High dose EHDP for prolonged periods of time appeared to retard mineralization of newly formed bone at active pagetic sites to the degree that some patients developed an increase in fractures. Moderate dose EHDP, 5 mg/kg/day, administered over 2 years, did not cause these effects. The current recommended dose in most patients is 5 mg/kg/day for 6 months. Therapy is stopped for a minimum of 3 months, but it can be restarted if necessary.

A third and less commonly used agent is the RNA-inhibiting mithramycin, derived from *Streptomyces plicatus.* It is a cytotoxic compound used in the treatment of various tumors. Because of its observed effect on calcium metabolism, the drug has been tried by Ryan and coworkers in Paget's disease (4). Lowering of serum calcium and relief of bone pain, which followed, encouraged these investigators to pursue its use in other patients. In a later study the treatment was found to be effective in 55 patients. Immediate, often "dramatic," subjective improvement paralleled objective evidence of suppressed disease activity, such as marked reduction of serum alkaline phosphatase and urinary hydroxyproline levels.

Repeated courses of therapy induced remissions in patients who tended to relapse. In those with localized disease, additional x-ray treatment enhanced the therapeutic benefit. Bone biopsy showing a decrease in osteoclasts, as well as in vitro studies with ^{45}Ca and hydroxyproline tagged with ^{14}C, suggested that the drug exerts its effect primarily through destruction of osteoclasts responsible for excessive bone resorption. Inhibition of bone resorption by mithramycin may not, however, be its sole beneficial action. Long-term therapy is essentially precluded by the drug's toxicity. Side effects during therapy are common.

Mithramycin is administered intravenously, 15 to 25 mg/kg/day for 10 days. It is frequently advisable to supplement the intravenous with a calcium salt as hypocalcimia is common. Mithramycin has also been used in conjunction with diphosphonates.

REFERENCES

1. Paget J. On a form of chronic inflammation of bones (osteitis) deformans. Med Chir Trans London 60:37, 1877.
2. Barry HC. Paget's Disease of Bone. Baltimore: Williams & Wilkins, 1970.
3. Singer ER, Fredericks RS, Minkin C. Salmon calcitonin therapy for Paget's disease of bone. Arthritis Rheum 23:1148–1154, 1980.
4. Ryan WG, Schwartz TB. Mithramycin treatment of Paget's disease of bone. Arthritis Rheum 23:1155–1161, 1980.
5. Khairi MRA, Johnston CC Jr, Altman RD, Willman HN, Serafini AN, Sanbey RR. Treatment of Paget's disease of bone (osteitus deformans). Results of a one-year study with sodium etidronate. JAMA 130:562, 1980.
6. Johnston CC Jr, Khairi RA, Meunier PJ. Use of etidronate (EHDP) in Paget's disease of bone. Arthritis Rheum 23:1172–1176, 1980.

TOTAL JOINT REPLACEMENT

JOHN J. JENNINGS, M.D.

A total joint replacement may be defined as the resurfacing of a diseased diarthrodial, or movable, joint by resection of the damaged cartilaginous surfaces and the insertion of an inert metal or plastic prosthetic device. Such devices have been developed over the past 25 years by orthopaedic surgeons. However, it was not until the past decade that their practical application has been realized. A major problem with such prostheses is the manner in which they are fixed to the underlying bone. Many previous prostheses developed loosening with the stresses of function and became painful.

Methyl methacrylate, an acrylic cement, has been used in the human body since the 1940s by neurosurgeons to repair skull defects. It has been well tolerated and has not been shown to be carcinogenic. Presently, it is used to bond mechanically the prostheses to bone surfaces. It is used in a puttylike state that is a mixture of a liquid monomer and a powder polymer. It sets rapidly into a rock-hard cement. The major toxicity in its use is that the monomer may be absorbed at the time of insertion and can act as a peripheral vasodilator. Death due to hypotensive crises has been reported. Such a problem can be avoided by an informed anesthesiologist.

Indications for total joint replacement are pain not controlled by nonsurgical means and loss of function of that joint. Nonsurgical means must include not only appropriate medications but rest of the entire body or of the specific joint with the use of external supports such as canes, crutches, and walkers. Total joint replacement is only indicated if more conservative surgery will not provide a painless and functional joint. Active sepsis of the involved joint is an absolute contraindication to joint replacement. The problem of total joint replacement in a joint previously infected but now quiescent is unresolved. The decision to replace such a joint can only be made after thorough medical evaluation, aspiration, and bone and soft tissue scanning. Youth is a relative contraindication in that the device, if stressed, will wear out eventually. The rapidity of wear has not yet been defined precisely since it is a function of prosthetic design, patient size, patient activity, and surgical technique. Data are available for wear in total hip replacements for 10 years. Wear over a decade seems minimal. The definitive answer will come only with longer experience.

The greatest problem in total joint replacement for the lower extremity is loosening. Since the acrylic cement only acts in a mechanical manner, it is the weak link in the system. With repeated cyclic loading, the cement has been shown to break down; eventually the entire prosthesis loosens. Various new designs are available on an experimental basis that no longer use methyl methacrylate cement. Such devices are coated with a porous type material that permits bony ingrowths into the surface of the prosthesis. If this can be accomplished in a uniform manner, the prosthesis will be well fixed without the use of cement.

There are multiple designs for joint replacements for all major joints. This portends that none is ideal for all clinical situations. It is necessary that a system of prosthetic designs be present in the operating room so that the device fits the patient, rather than the patient being made to fit the device.

The current materials used to manufacture joint replacement protheses are inert metals (high grade stainless steel, chrome cobalt alloys, and, more recently, titanium alloys), ultrahigh molecular weight polyethylene, and surgical grade silastic. Such materials are well tolerated by the body and have not yet been shown to evoke either an immunologic or a carcinogenic response.

TOTAL HIP REPLACEMENT

Total hip replacement is indicated in many affections of the hip joint, including idiopathic osteoarthritis, rheumatoid arthritis, avascular necrosis, psoriatic arthritis, congenital hip dysplasia, traumatic arthritis, and, rarely, such entities as tumors (both primary and metastatic), fractures, and pseudogout.

There are many satisfactory prosthetic designs available that have the common feature of a metallic sphere with an intramedullary stem moving against a high density polyethylene socket.

Technically, after resection of the diseased femoral head, the acetabulum is first deepened and roughened for the cementing in of the socket. Once the socket is in place, the femoral canal is reamed for the insertion of the cemented femoral component stem. Formerly, it was customary to detach the greater trochanter for exposure's sake and then reattach it to the femoral shaft at the end of the case. Currently, most total hip replacements can be done without trochanteric osteotomy. This negates the complications of trochanteric nonunion and fracturing of the wires.

Most total hip replacement patients recover rapidly and are ambulatory in the first few days. However, patients are usually required to use some type of external support (e.g., crutches or a cane) for several months. The postoperative results evaluated by one of many hip rating scales show good to excellent surgical results in more than 90% of patients. No other reconstructive hip operation gives such a predictable, high level of good results. Many patients with severe bilateral hip arthritides have received bilateral hip replacements during the same hospitalization with dramatic relief of pain. This surgery must be done by an orthopaedic surgeon who is trained in this type of operation. It is an excellent procedure but not a panacea. These patients, although able to resume full activity, do not have a normal joint. Such patients should be cautioned against any activities that rapidly and cyclically load the hip such as jogging, running, and playing competitive sports.

SURFACE REPLACEMENT OF THE HIP JOINT

In the past 5 years, a newer surgical procedure has become moderately popular and has met with modest success. This procedure is a surface replacement of the hip. Its attractiveness lies in the fact that the femoral head is not sacrificed and the joint is merely resurfaced by placing a thin polyethylene shell into the acetabulum and a thin metallic cup over the femoral head. At this writing, the procedure has only been done and followed in significant numbers for a short period of time. In several series, the complication rate is much higher than that in total hip replacement, so the procedure must be viewed as experimental.

TOTAL KNEE REPLACEMENT

Much of the technical knowledge gained from total hip replacement has been applicable to the replacement of other joints. Total knee replacements usually refer to the resurfacing of the femoral condyles and tibial plateaus. Recently the patellofemoral articulation has been surgically replaced. There are now prosthetic devices that resurface the patella, but their efficacy has not yet stood the test of time.

The earlier total knee prostheses were of the metallic hinge-type and met with limited success. The use of methyl methacrylate for better fixation has enhanced the results. However, if the knee is analyzed biomechanically, it is evident that it is not a simple hinge. Along with the hinge arc of motion, there is sliding, gliding, and rotation of the tibia on the femur. Articulated prostheses of metal-against-plastic design have been developed to permit such motion. The prime indication for their use is the relief of pain in knees not amenable to medical or more conservative surgical management. Active pyogenic sepsis is a contraindication. Since the articulated devices depend on the soft tissue for stability, they are used mainly in knees that are relatively stable and do not have gross deformity. The hinge device is best limited to patients with marked deformity and instability. Although the hip replacement patient requires postoperative physical therapy, it is not of the degree necessary in the knee replacement patient who must do regular intensive exercises in order to maximize the quality of the surgical result.

A biomechanical approach to the knee joint with the design of anametric devices has markedly enhanced the success in these procedures. The earlier articulated prostheses almost universally with several years of use began to show loosening of the tibial component with the appearance of a radiolucent line in the bone cement interface of the tibia. Many of these, subsequently, went on to become clinically loose and painful. Such has not been the case with the newer prostheses, and it is a realistic hope that their longevity will equal that of the total hip replacements.

HAND JOINT REPLACEMENT

Metacarpophalangeal (MCP) joint replacement is used almost exclusively in the rheumatoid arthritic patient with destruction of the MCP joint and subsequent pain and loss of function. The devices are hingelike in design and serve to stabilize the joint and permit painless but meaningful motion. Most are made of silastic, an inert rubberlike material. The patients often have severe deformity. Postoperatively they do not have normal functioning hands, but they are better able to carry out the activities of daily living in greater comfort.

Probably in no other surgical procedure is the demand for long-lasting and intense postoperative therapy as great as it is in hand joint replacement. These patients must be willing to participate actively and intensively in their therapy under good direction if a surgical success is to be attained. This often will take many months of post-operative splinting and exercise under the care of a well-trained hand therapist.

OTHER JOINTS

Much active research is being conducted in the field of joint replacement. Devices are available for use in the elbow, ankle, shoulder, wrist, and temporomandibular joints. Their success is not yet established.

Successful joint replacement is directly dependent on patient selection, surgical technique, and postoperative management. Only if all three are of excellent quality will the result be comparable.

INDEX

A

Acute dermatomyositis-polymyositis (AD-P), 112–117
  in children, 116
  clinical features, 114–116
  interstitial fibrosis, 113
  laboratory findings, 116–117
  malignancy, 112, 116
  pathogenesis, 112–113
  pathology, 113
  prognosis, 117
  treatment, 117
Acute rheumatic fever (ARF), 136–140
  clinical course, 138
  clinical features, 137
  diagnosis, 138
  epidemiology, 136
  Jones criteria for diagnosis, 138
  laboratory findings, 138–139
  pathogenesis, 136–137
  recurrence, prevention of, 140
  treatment, 139–140
Alkaptonuria, in ochronosis, 193
Allele, 25
Allopurinol (Zyloprim), 160
Alopecia, 104
Alternative pathway, complement system, 1, 3, 6–8
  components of, 1
  regulation of, 7–8
Altman, Roy D., 102–111; 123–129; 141–145; 190–192; 198–206
American Rheumatism Association, criteria for classification,
  rheumatoid arthritis, 51–52
  systemic lupus erythematosus (SLE), 102–105
Anaphylatoxin inactivator, 2
Ankylosing spondylitis (AS), 73–78
  aspirin, 77
  characteristics of, 73
  clinical course, 77
  clinical findings, 73–76
  dorsal kyphosis, 75
  erythrocyte sedimentation rate, 76
  exercises, 77
  family incidence, 73
  laboratory findings, 76–77
  poker spine, 75
  symptoms, 73
  therapy, 77–78
Antinuclear antibodies (ANA), 21–24; 109
  classes, 22
  Crithidia technique, 109
  Farr technique, 109
  fluorescent staining, 23–24
  testing, 22–23
Arachidonic acid, 32–34

Arthralgias and SLE, 105
Arthritis mutilans, 80
Arthritis without deformity, 104–105
Arthropathy, secondary degenerative, 190–191
Autosome, 25

B

Backache, low, 181–183
  cause, 181, 182
  incidence of, 181
  psychogenic disorders, 182
  rheumatoid variants, 182
  spondylosis, 182
  tension rheumatism, 182
  therapy, 183
Baker's cysts, 99
Blechman, Wilbur J., 66–72; 184–186
Brown, Harvey E., 73–78; 85–86
Bursitis, 184–185
  anserine, 185
  calcaneal, 185
  ischial, 184
  subdeltoid, 184
  treatment, 186
  trochanteric, 185
  Weaver's bottom, 184
Butterfly rash, 103

C

Calcium pyrophosphate arthropathy, *see* Pseudogout
Calcium pyrophosphate dihydrate (CPPD) crystals, 47
Caplan's syndrome, 58
Carpal tunnel syndrome, 185
  in rheumatoid arthritis, 53
Cartilage, pathophysiology, 163, 171
  articular cartilage, 170
  cartilage matrix, uniqueness of, 170
  chondryocyte territory, 170
  collagen, 166–170
  osteoarthritis pathology, inflammatory component, 170–171
  proteoglycan, 163–165
Cellular casts, 105
Chondrocalcinosis, 187–189
  crystal deposition, 188
  in other diseases, 187
  pseudogout, 187
  secondary, 191
  treatment, 188–189
  U.S., form, 187
Chondrocytes, 165, 170
Chronic false-positive STS, 105
Chrysotherapy, 35
  rheumatoid arthritis, 62–63
Classic pathway, complement system, 1, 4–6
  components, 1
  native C3 activation and cleavage, 4
  receptor sites, 5
Collagen, 166–170
  breakdown, 169–170
  formation, 167–168
  hydroxyproline, 166–157
  rheumatoid arthritis, 170
  synthesis and assembly, 166–167
  triple helix, 168
Complement assays, clinical application of, 8–9
  C quantification, 9
  connective tissue disorders, 8
  hypocomplementemia, 9
  immunofluorescent studies, 8
Complement deficiency states, 9–11
  genetic abnormalities, 10
  literature review, 9–10
Complement system and inflammation, 1–19
  alternative pathway, 1, 3, 6–8
  anaphylatoxic fragments, 2
  bradykinin, 2
  C1 esterase inhibitor, 11–12

C1q, 12–13
C1r, 13
C1s, 13
C2, 13–14
C3, 14
C3b inactivator, 14
C4, 13
C5 functional and protein defects, 15
C6, 15
C7, 15–16
C8, 16
classic pathway, 1, 4–6
complement assays, 8–9
complement deficiency states, 9–11
immunoglobulins, 2–3
inactivators, 1
inhibitors, 1
Convulsions and SLE, 105
Coombs' positive hemolytic anemia in SLE, 107
Corticosteroids
acute rheumatic fever, 139
mixed connective tissue disease, 131
osteoarthritis, 178
polymyalgia rheumatic, 134–135
rheumatoid arthiritis, 63
SLE, 110, 111
Cryoglobulinemia, 86
Cytotaxic agents in SLE, 111

D

Degenerative joint disease synovianalysis, 49
DeQuervain's disease, 185
Discoid lupus erythematosus (DLE), 102, 103

E

Eosinophilic fasciitis, 132–133
laboratory studies, 133
recurrences, 133
symptoms, 132
Erythema chronicum migrans (ECM), 98
treatment, 100–101
Evan's syndrome in SLE, 107

F

Facial erythema, 103
Factor XI, 30
Factor XII activated system, 28–31
action mechanisms, 30–31
amino acid sequence, 30
forms of, 28–29
kiminogen, 28
substances that activate, 28
substrates, 29–30
Felty's syndrome, 83–84
laboratory studies, 83
pyoderma gangrenosum, 84
spleen, 83
treatment, 84
Fibrositis, 186
Fletcher factor, 30

G

Genotype, 25
Gonococcal arthritis (GC), 141–145
Center for Disease Control, recommended therapy for disseminated gonococcal infection, 144
clinical manifestations, 141–142
laboratory findings, 143
Neisseria gonorrhoeae, 143
pregnancy, 143
treatment, 143–144
Gottlieb, Norman L., 41–50; 51–65; 87–92; 93–97; 98–101; 118–122; 193–197
Gout
patients, 147
synovianalysis, 46–47
Gout and hyperuricemia, 152–162
Allopurinol (Zyloprim), 160
asymptomatic hyperuricemia, 161–162

Gout and hyperuricemia [cont.]
- blood pressure elevation, 159
- clinical features, 153–154
- colchicine therapy, 156–157; 159–161
- complications, 158–159
- course, 158
- diagnosis, 156–158
- diet, 161
- great toe involvement, 153
- idiopathic hyperuricemia, 155–156
- laboratory findings, 155
- podagra, 153
- precipitating agents, 154
- primary gout, 152
- Probenecid (Benemid), 160
- purine biosynthesis, 152
- secondary gout, 152–153
- serum uric acid elevation, 157
- severe chronic tophaceous gout, 156
- treatment, 159–161
- urate stones, 158–159
- uric acid crystals in synovial fluid, 156

H

Hageman factor, 28–31. *See also* Factor XII activated systems
Hand joint replacement, 210–211
Haplotype, 25
Hemochromatosis, 190–192
- ostepenia, 191
- secondary chondrocalcinosis, 191
- secondary degenerative arthropathy, 190–191

Hemolytic anemia and SLE, 105
Henoch-Shoenlein appearing purpura, 108
Hepatitis, 93-94
Histocompatibility antigens (HLA), 24–26
- in diseases, 25–26
- LD, 25
- SD, 25

Hip replacement
- external supports, 209
- surface replacement, 209
- total, 208–209

Howell, David S., 79–82; 83–84; 172–180; 181–183; 187–189
Hyer, Fred H., 93–97
Hypergammaglobulinemia in SLE, 108
Hyperuricemia, 150–151
- asymptomatic, 161–162
- and gout, 151–162. *See also* Gout
- hypoxanthine-guanine phosphoribosyltransferase (HG-PRTase), 151
- idiopathic, 155–156

Hypocomplementemia, 9

I

Immune response (Ir) genes, 25
Immunogenetics. *See* Complement deficiency states
Immunoglobulins, 2–3
Immunosuppressive agents in SLE, 110
Inflammation and complement system, 1–19. *See also* Complement system
Inflammatory process, mediators of, 28–40
- antigen-antibody complexes, 36
- antiinflammatory drugs, 34–35
- arachidonic acid oxidation products, 32–34
- chrysotherapy, 35
- copper, 35
- factor XII activated systems, 28–31
- glucocorticoids, 35
- leukotrienes, 33
- lysosomal enzymes, 35–37
- PG of E group, 34
- PMN leukocytes, 36

prostacyclin PGL_2, 32
prostaglandins, 31–32
thromboxanes, 32
Ixodes damini, 98

J
Jennings, John J., 207–211
Joint aspiration technique, 41–42
aseptic technique, 41
latrogenic joint infection, 42
Joint replacement. *See* Total joint replacement
Jones criteria for guidance in diagnosis of rheumatic fever (1973), 138
Juvenile rheumatoid arthritis. *See* Rheumatoid arthritis, juvenile

K
Keratoderma blennorrhagica, 89
Knee replacement, total, 210
Koebner phenomenon, 66

L
LE cells, 105
Lesch-Nyhan syndrome, 151
Leukopenia and SLE, 105, 107
Linkage of genes, 25
Locus of gene, 25
Lyme disease (LD), 98–101
age of onset, 98
antibiotics for, 100–101
clinical manifestations, 98–100
erythema chronicum migrans (ECM), 98
geographic clustering of cases, 98
Ixodes dammini, 98
laboratory data, 100
pathogenesis, 98
treatment, 100–101
Lymphadenopathy, 67

M
Major histocompatibility complex (MHC), 25
Medrol for SLE, 111
Metacarpophalangeal (MCP) joint replacement, 210–211
Methylprenisolone acetate for SLE, 111
Mixed connective tissue (MCTD), 130–131
clinical features, 130–131
treatment and prognosis, 131
Mucin clot, 44
Mumps, 95
Mycoplasma, 95

O
Ochronosis, 193–197
alkaptonuria, 193
clinical findings, 193–196
etiology, 193
homogentisic acid oxidase absence, 193
pathology, 196
spondylosis, 194–195
treatment, 196
Oral or nasopharyngeal ulceration, 104
Osteoarthritis (OA), 172–180
articular cartilage, 174–175
biochemical studies, 175–176
clinical findings, 177
corticosteroids, 178
definitions and incidence, 172–173
Kellgren, 173
management, 177
medical measures, 177–178
microtrauma, 176–177
nutrition therapy, 177
pathogenesis, 176–177
pathology and phsyiology, 174–176
physical therapy, 178–179
primary, 173

Osteoarthritis (OA) [cont.]
salicylates, 178
secondary, 173
surgical intervention, 179
Osteoarthritis pathology, inflammatory component, International Symposium, 170–171
Osteopenia, 191

P

Paget's disease, 198–206
clinical features, 202
diagnosis, 203
disodium etidronate (EHDP) (Didronel), 204
mithramycin, 206
pathology and pathophysiology, 198–201
pyrophosphate, 204–205
remissions, 205
salicylates, 203
signs of, 202
streptomyces plicatus, 205
synthetic salmon calcitonin (Calcimar), 204
treatment, 203–206
Paraamino benzoic acid (POTABA) and scleroderma, 128
Penicillin
acute rheumatic fever, 139
gonococcal arthritis, 143
rheumatoid arthritis, 63
Pericarditis and SLE, 105
Peripheral asymmetric polyarthritis, 79–80
Phagocytosis, 36
Phenotype, 25
Photosensitivity, 104
Pita, Julio C., 147–151
Plasma thromboplastin antecedent, 30
Plasminogen proactivator, 30, 31
Pleuritis and SLE, 105
Podagra, 153
Polyarteritis nodusa (PAN), 118–122
clinical manifestations, 118–122
course and treatment, 121
diagnosis, 121
etiology, 118
laboratory tests, 120
Polymyalgia rheumatica, 134–135
clinical features, 134
therapy, 134–135
Polymyositis. *See* Acute dermatomyositis polymyositis
Prekallikren activator (PKA), 29
Probenecid (Benemid), 160
Profuse proteinuria, 105
Progressive systemic sclerosis. *See* Scleroderma
Properdin pathway. *See* Alternative pathway, complement system
Prostacyclin (PGL_2), 32
Prostaglandins, 31–32
Proteoglycan, 163–165
aggregate pathology, 164–165
anionic aggregate, 164
chondrocytes, 165
enzymes, 165
monomer, 163, 164
side chains, 163
Pseudogout, 187
synovianalysis, 47
Psoriatic arthritis, 79–82
antiinflammatory drugs, 82
arthritis mutilans, 80
azathioprine (Imuran), 82
course of disease, 80
histocompatibility laboratory test (HLA-B27), 81
peripheral asymmetric polyarthritis, 79–80
radiologic features, 81–82
reconstructive surgery, 82
sausage fingers or toes, 80
treatment, 82
Psychosis and SLE, 105

Purine metabolism, 147–151
- Allopurinol (Zyloprim), 151
- amidotransferase, 148
- gout patients, 147
- hyperuricemia, 150–151
- inosinic acid (IMP), 149
- purine biosynthesis, 152
- purine ring formation, 147–148
- regulatory control, 149
- uric acid, 147

Pyoderma gangrenosum, 84

R

Raynaud's phenomenon
- and scleroderma, 123–124
- and SLE, 103

Reiter's syndrome (RS), 87–92
- clinical features, 87–90
- course and treatment, 91
- heart disease, 90
- histocompatibility antigen B27, 91
- keratoderma blennorrhagica, 89
- laboratory findings, 90–91
- ocular involvement, 88–89
- presentation, 87
- severity and duration, 88
- skin involvement, 89
- synovianalysis, 47–48

Relaxin and scleroderma, 128

Rheumatoid arthritis (RA), 51–65
- acute phase phenomenon, 61
- American Rheumatism Association criteria, 51–52
- anemia, 60
- blood elements, 60
- Caplan's syndrome, 58
- cardiac involvement, 57–58
- clinical features, 53–56
- chloroquine, 62
- chrysotherapy, 62–63
- corticosteroids, 63
- cytotoxic agents, 63–64
- entrapment neuropathies, 54
- epidemiology, 51–52
- extraarticular features, 56–60
- histidine, 63
- hydroxychloroquine, 62
- immune factors, 61
- incidence, 51–52
- laboratory tests, 60–61
- Levamisole, 64
- liver function, 61
- medical synovectomy, 64
- neurologic manifestations, 59
- ocular findings, 58
- penicillamine, 63
- reconstructive orthopedic surgery, 64
- renal function, 61
- secondary amyloidosis, 60
- skin involvement, 59–60
- subluxation, 54–55
- surgical synovectomy, 64
- swan-neck deformity, 55
- synovianalysis, 48
- synovial membrane, 51
- systemic or malignant, 56
- treatment, 61–64

Rheumatoid arthritis, juvenile, 66–72
- antinuclear antibodies (ANA), 68–69
- classification, 66
- diagnosis, 71
- incidence, 66–67
- mode of onset, 70
- presentations, 66–71
- slit-lamp examination, 69
- therapy, 71–72
- Tolmetin, 71

Rheumatoid factors (RE), 20–21
- as activator of effector systems, 21
- antigamma globulin, 20
- defined, 20
- detection of, 20
- in rheumatoid arthritis, 21

Ropes' test, 44

Rubella, 94

S

Salicylates
  acute rheumatic fever, 139
  osteoarthritis, 178
  Paget's disease, 203
  SLE, 110
Sarcoidosis, 146
Sausage fingers or toes, 80
Schirmer filter paper test, 86
Schultz, Duane R., 1–19; 20–27; 28–40
Scleroderma, 123–129
  claw hand, 124
  clinical features, 123–127
  course, 128
  diagnosis, 128
  gastrointestinal tract involvement, 125–126
  laboratory findings, 128
  microvascularitis, 126
  pathogenesis, 123
  Raynaud's phenomenon, 123–124
  renal involvement, 126–127
  skin involvement, 125
  therapy, 128–129
Secondary osteoarthritis, 173. *See also* Osteoarthritis
Septic arthritis
  synovianalysis, 49
Serology, 20–27
  antinuclear antibodies (ANA), 21–24
  histocompatibility antigens (HLA), 24–26
  rheumatoid factors (RE), 20–21
Sjögren's syndrome, 85–86
  cryoglobulinemia, 86
  incidence, 85
  neuromuscular abnormalities, 86
  Schirmer filter paper test, 86
  sicca complex, 85
  symptoms, 85
  treatment, 86
Smallpox, 95
Synovianalysis, 41–50
  in calcium pyrophosphate arthropathy (pseudogout), 47
  counting chamber, 44
  degenerative joint disease, 49
  gout, 46–47
  joint aspiration, 41–42
  microscopic examination, 45
  mucin clot, 44
  normal synovial fluid, 43–44
  Reiter's syndrome, 47–48
  rheumatoid arthritis, 48
  rheumatoid factor, 45
  results of, 42–43
  septic arthritis, 49
  synovial fluid examination, 44–46
  traumatic arthritis, 48–49
Systemic lupus erythematosus (SLE), 102–111
  antinuclear antibodies (ANA), 109
  arthralgias, 105
  cardiac involvement, 106
  diagnosis, 102–105
  drug-induced, 108, 109
  emotional stress, 108
  family studies, controlled, 108
  hair loss, 108
  hematologically, 107
  immunologic mechanisms, 108
  kidneys, 106
  lung, 106
  mortality associated with, 109–110
  nervous system, 106
  ocular findings, 107
  prognosis, 109–110
  protein abnormalities, 108–109
  skin involvement, 107–108
  sunlight exposure, 108
  symptoms, 105–106
  syndrome, 105–109
  therapy, 110–111

T

Talbott, John H., 112–117; 130–131; 132–133; 134–135; 136–140; 146; 152–162
Tendonitis, 185–186
  bicipital, 185
  carpal tunnel syndrome, 185
  DeQuervain's disease, 185
  tennis elbow, 185
  treatment, 186
  trigger fingers, 186
Tennis elbow, 185
Tenosynovitis, 53
  digital flexor, 54
Thrombocytopenia and SLE, 105, 107
Thromboxanes, 32
Total joint replacement, 207–211
  defined, 207
  designs, 208
  hand, 210–211
  indications for, 207
  knee, 210
  materials, 208
  methyl methacrylate, 207
  patient selection, 211
  postoperative management, 211
  problems, 208
  surface hip replacement, 209
  technique, 211
  total hip replacement, 208–209
Tophaceous gout, severe chronic, 156
Traumatic arthritis
  synovianalysis, 48–49
Trigger fingers, 185

U

Unschuld, Hal B., 98–101

V

Varicella-zoster, 94–95
Viral arthritis, 93–97
  acute tropical polyarthritis, 96
  EB virus, 96
  echo virus type 9 infection, 96
  erythema infectiosum, 96
  hepatitis, 93–94
  monoarticulor, 96
  mumps, 95
  mycoplasma, 95
  associated with respiratory syndrome, 96
  rubella, 94
  smallpox, 95
  varicella-zoster, 94–95

W

Weaver's bottom, 184
Woessner, J.F., 163–171